101 Fat-Burning
Workouts & Diet Strategies

Acknowledgments

This publication is based on articles written by Chris Aceto, Jeanine Detz, Jon Finkel, Bill Geiger, Matthew G. Kadey, Peter McGough, Jimmy Peña, Carey Rossi, Jim Stoppani, PhD, Mark Thorpe, Eric Velazquez and Joe Wuebben.

Cover photography by Michael Darter.

Photography by Per Bernal, Art Brewer, Charles Imstepf Studios, Michael Darter, Kevin Horton, Iconmen.com, Naj Jamai, Blake Little, Ian Logan, Geoffrey Nicholson, Joaquin Palting, Robert Reiff, Marc Royce, Ian Spanier, Brian Velenchenko and Pavel Ythjall.

Project editor is Michael Berg, NSCA-CPT.

Project managing editor is Vicki Baker.

Project copy editors are Erin Newman and James Riley.

Project design by Michael Touna and KiWon Ballman.

Photo assistant is Amina Cruz.

Editor in Chief/Group Editorial Director of *Muscle & Fitness* is Peter McGough.
Founding Chairman is Joe Weider. Chairman and CEO of American Media, Inc., is David Pecker.

ISBN: 978-1-60078-205-3

Printed in USA.

PRESENTED BY **MUSCLE & FITNESS** MAGAZINE

101 Fat-Burning
Workouts & Diet Strategies

TRIUMPH
BOOKS

MICHAEL BERG, NSCA-CPT
AND THE EDITORS OF *MUSCLE & FITNESS*

Contents

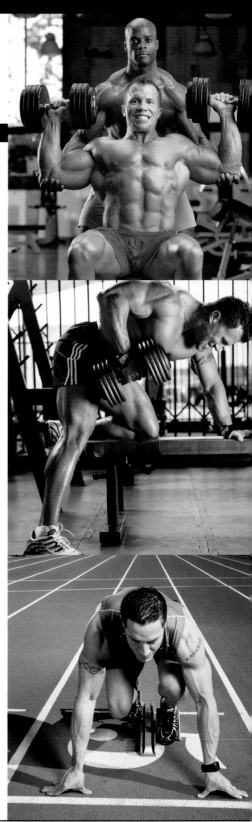

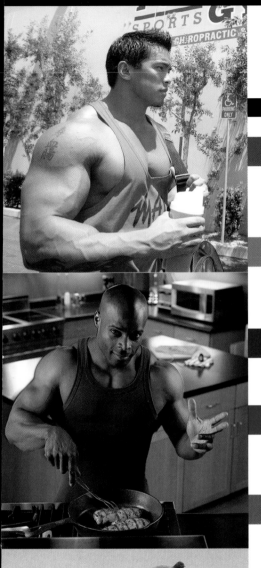

SECTION TWO NUTRITION

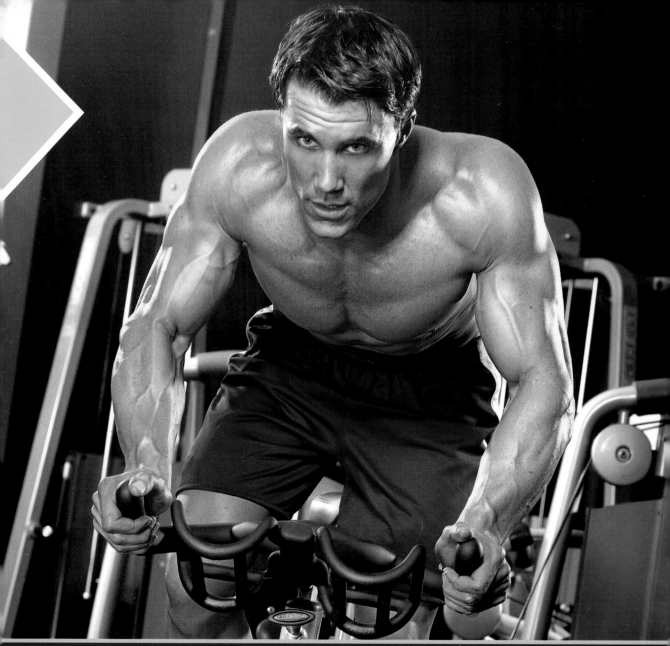

SECTION ONE
TRAIN

The quest for your best-ever body begins here. In the following pages, you'll find an incredible compendium of workout routines, effective exercises and fat-searing cardio options all designed with one overriding goal in mind: To help you lean out while also getting fitter and more muscular at the same time. Turn the page to get started.

ING

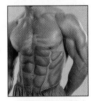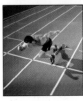

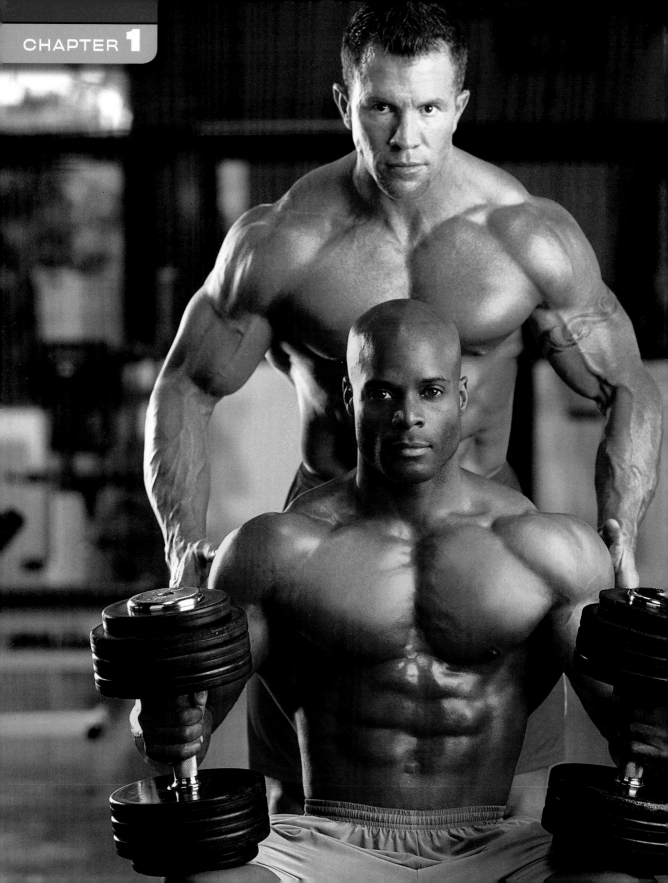

Ultimate Training Guide

We've all been there. In general, your workouts have never been better, but those pesky lower lats are about as responsive as a tackle dummy Or maybe your outer quads or front delts are more Gary Coleman than Ronnie Coleman and just refuse to grow. Then again, perhaps the problem is your entire pec area, or you sport hams that are more like Spam — soft and far from the real thing. Or it could be you're just pressed for time and want to know how to perform a decent back workout in just 15 minutes.

Cue "Workout Central," your one-stop shop for muscle size, strength and definition. In this chapter, we offer 86 workouts, one or more of which we can virtually guarantee will solve your individual training problems. You'd be hard-pressed to find this many individual routines so easy to navigate in one place.

In addition, we provide an efficient 40-minute, total-body workout plan designed especially for those balancing a great physique with a hectic schedule, plus targeted advice for gaining overall muscle mass or getting super lean. So what are you waiting for? Identify your problem, look up the solution and start turning a weakness into a strength.

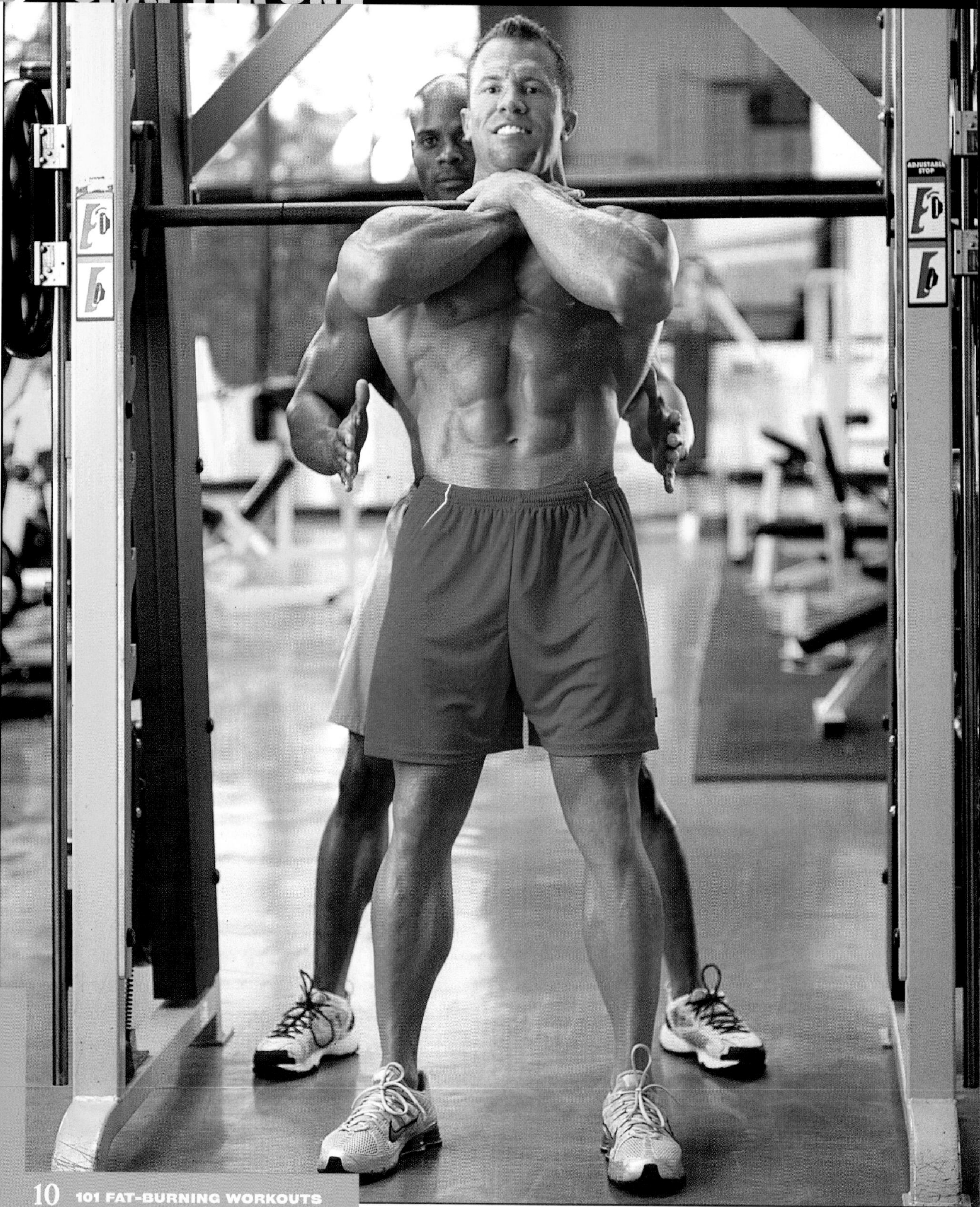
ADJUSTABLE STOP

ROUTINE KEY

THROUGHOUT THE FOLLOWING PAGES, YOU'LL FIND NUMEROUS ROUTINES THAT ADDRESS DIFFERENT TRAINING GOALS AND TROUBLE SPOTS. HERE'S A QUICK GUIDE TO THOSE CATEGORIES AND WHAT THEY ENTAIL.

>> **MASS-BUILDING** ROUTINE
Compound movements, high volume and moderate rep ranges for maximizing muscle growth.

>> **BEGINNER'S** ROUTINE
Mostly machine-based exercises for those still getting their feet wet before progressing to more advanced moves.

>> **AT-HOME** ROUTINE
Requires nothing more than dumbbells and an adjustable bench, a common home-gym setup.

>> **15-MINUTE WORKOUT** ROUTINE
Short rest periods and multiple exercises using minimal equipment for a faster pace. (For abs, we offer a 10-minute routine instead of 15.)

>> **"PRIORITY" WORKOUT** ROUTINE
For targeting a specific area of a muscle that needs to be brought up. A priority workout will train other areas of the muscle as well (for example, the short head of the biceps will also be worked in the long head priority workout), just not to the extent of the intended location.

>> **GIANT-SET** ROUTINE
All exercises are done consecutively without resting between sets to achieve ultrahigh intensity.

>> **STRENGTH** ROUTINE
Lower reps, heavier weight and longer rest periods for when pure strength and power are priorities.

>> **GET RIPPED** ROUTINE
High volume, high reps and short rest periods to increase intensity and boost metabolism for greater fat-burning potential.

>> **GET SUPER PUMPED** ROUTINE
High reps and short rest periods for increased blood flow to muscles.

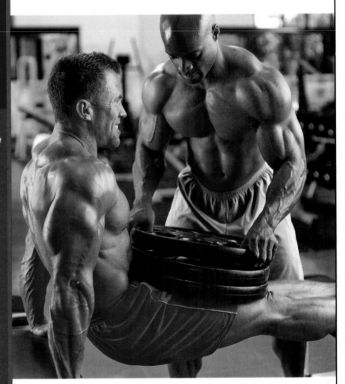

MAKE IT WORK FOR YOU

This chapter is designed to help anyone construct a workout specifically for his needs. In the list at left, you'll see all of the various types of training sessions we provide for all of the major bodyparts.

Here's how to use it. Say your goal is to pack more muscle onto a skinny frame. Just pick out all of the "mass-building routines" and assemble them into one training split — you could do chest and triceps on Monday, back and bi's on Tuesday, thighs and calves on Thursday, and delts, traps, forearms (and abs) on Friday. Same advice goes if you're after more strength — pull out all the "strength" workouts and design a weekly split that works within your schedule.

Of course, you don't have to completely revamp your current workout routine, if you have one. You can use the following workouts as replacements for one or more bodypart-focused routines, as a way to freshen up a stale regimen. You can even pick out a few new exercises and insert them into existing workouts. The options are limited only by your imagination.

BACK

When targeting a specific area of a muscle, exercise selection is key. In the lower lats priority workout, the movements (most notably back exercises performed using a narrow reverse grip, including the chin) are all effective at zeroing in on the lower portion of the lats, which, when fully developed, create a more dramatic V-taper. In the upper lats priority workout, all exercises are done with a wide overhand grip, which helps develop back width just below the armpits. Ideally you'd utilize both underhand and overhand grips in a given back workout, but each of the aforementioned routines are great for bringing up their respective areas when a weakness is present.

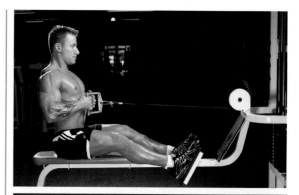

Seated Row

» Attach a close-grip handle to a row apparatus and sit upright on the bench facing the weight stack. Place your feet on the platform, legs slightly bent. Reach forward to grasp the handle; keep your back flat and chest up. With your torso erect, arms fully extended, pull the handle toward your midsection. Keep your elbows in, your torso erect and your head in a neutral position. Squeeze your back muscles. Hold for 1-2 seconds before slowly returning to the start position.

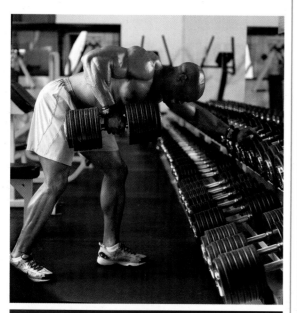

Dumbbell Row

» Bend at the waist, placing one knee and the same-side hand on a flat bench (or lean into a sturdy rack). If using a bench, keep your other foot on the floor beside it and hold a dumbbell in the same-side hand, arm fully extended down. Pull the weight toward your hip, bringing your elbow up as high as you can, keeping it close to you. Squeeze your shoulder blades together, then lower the weight along the same path. Repeat for reps, then switch arms.

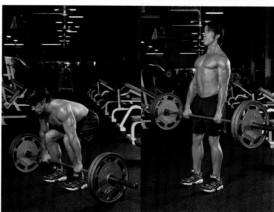

Deadlift

» Feet flat under a bar, squat down and take a slightly wider than shoulder-width grip. Allow the bar to rest against your shins. With your chest up and back flat, lift the bar by extending your hips and knees fully. Keep your arms straight throughout, as you drag the bar up your legs till you are in a standing position. Squeeze your back, legs and glutes, then lower the bar along the same path till it touches the floor. Allow the bar to settle before beginning the next rep.

#1 MASS-BUILDING

EXERCISE	SETS	REPS
Deadlift	5	6, 6, 8, 10, 12
Bent-Over Row	5	8, 8, 10, 10, 12
Seated Row	4	8, 8, 10, 12
Lat Pulldown	3	8, 10, 12

#2 BEGINNER'S

EXERCISE	SETS	REPS
Lat Pulldown	4	10, 10, 12, 12
Machine Row	3	10, 10, 10
Dumbbell Row	3	10, 10, 10
Standing Low-Cable Row	3	12, 12, 12

#3 AT-HOME

EXERCISE	SETS	REPS
Dumbbell Row	4	8, 10, 12, 20
Straight-Arm Kickback	4	10, 12, 12, 20
Pullover	4	8, 8, 12, 20

#4 15-MINUTE WORKOUT

EXERCISE	SETS[1]	REPS
Lat Pulldown	3	6, 10, 15
Reverse-Grip Pulldown	3	6, 10, 15
Seated Row	3	6, 10, 15

#5 LOWER LATS PRIORITY

EXERCISE	SETS	REPS
Reverse-Grip Bent-Over Row	4	10, 10, 12, 12
Close-Grip Lat Pulldown	4	8, 8, 10, 10
Straight-Arm Pulldown	3	10, 12, 15
Standing Low-Cable Row	3	10, 12, 15

#6 UPPER LATS PRIORITY

EXERCISE	SETS	REPS
Lat Pulldown	4	6, 10, 12, 15
Bent-Over Row	3	10, 10, 10
Wide-Grip Seated Row	3	8, 10, 12
Pull-Up	3	to failure

#7 GIANT-SET WORKOUT[2]

EXERCISE	SETS	REPS
Deadlift	4	10, 10, 10, 10
Bent-Over Row	4	10, 10, 10, 10
Rack Pull	4	10, 10, 10, 10
Pull-Up	4	to failure

#8 STRENGTH

EXERCISE	SETS[3]	REPS
Dumbbell Row	4	4, 4, 6, 8
Machine Row	4	4, 4, 6, 8
T-Bar Row	3	4, 6, 6
Seated Row	3	4, 6, 6

#9 GET RIPPED

EXERCISE	SETS[1]	REPS
Dumbbell Deadlift	5	10, 12, 12, 15, 20
Straight-Arm Pulldown	4	12, 12, 15, 15
Pullover	4	15, 15, 20, 20
Lat Pulldown	4	10, 12, 15, 20

#10 GET SUPER PUMPED

EXERCISE	SETS[1]	REPS
Bent-Over Row	4	10, 10, 30, 30
Seated Row	4	10, 10, 30, 30
Lat Pulldown	4	10, 10, 30, 30

[1] Rest no more than 30 seconds between each set.
[2] A giant set consists of four or more exercises performed consecutively without rest as a means to increase intensity and promote muscle growth. Do one set of each exercise back-to-back — that's one giant set. Rest three minutes between each giant set.
[3] Rest 2–3 minutes between each set.
Notes: The above workouts don't include warm-up sets. Unless otherwise noted, rest 60–90 seconds between all sets.

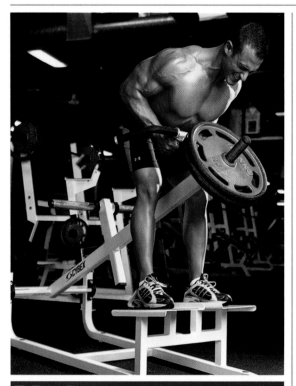

T-Bar Row

» With your arms fully extended, grasp the handles with an overhand, palms-forward grip. Wrap your thumbs around the bar for safety. Lift the bar upward, remaining in the bent-over position. Keep your chest up and back flat, head in a neutral position. Pull the handles toward you, keeping your elbows close to your body. Do not allow your upper body to raise in an effort to pull the weight upward. Hold the peak contracted position momentarily before slowly lowering the weight to the starting position.

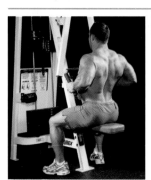

Machine Row

» Sit at a selectorized row machine, with your feet flat on the floor and your chest pressed against the pad. Grasp the handles with either a neutral or overhand grip, and pull the handles toward you, squeezing your lats briefly, then return to the start and repeat.

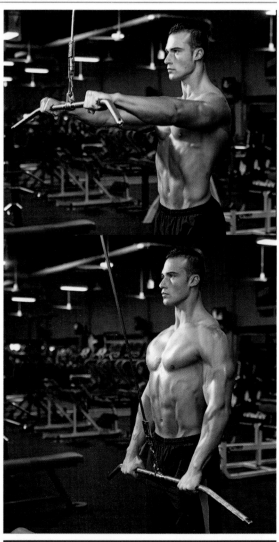

Straight-Arm Lat Pulldown

» Stand facing the weight stack at a lat-pulldown station with your feet shoulder-width apart. Reach up and grasp a standard lat-pulldown bar or long straight bar with an overhand (pronated) grip, hands shoulder-width apart, arms straight. Start with the bar at shoulder level, arms extended and parallel to the floor. Keeping your arms straight, pull the bar down toward your thighs in a wide, sweeping arc, focusing on using just your lats. Exhale as you pass the midpoint of the move, and squeeze your lats hard once the bar reaches your thighs. Return to the starting position in a smooth, controlled motion, stopping once your arms are parallel to the floor.

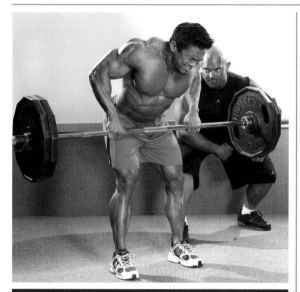

Bent-Over Row

» Standing with your feet shoulder–width apart, grasp a barbell with a wide, overhand grip. Keeping your knees slightly bent, lean forward at your waist until your torso is roughly parallel with the floor. The barbell should hang straight down in front of your shins. Without raising your upper body, pull the barbell up toward your abdomen, bringing your elbows high and above the level of your back. Hold the bar in the peak-contracted position for a brief count, then slowly lower along the same path. Repeat for reps.

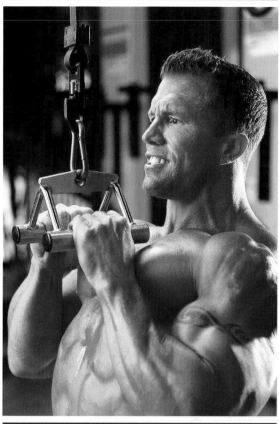

Close-Grip Pulldown

» Attach a V-bar to the pulley and adjust the kneepad so that you fit snugly in the seat. Grasp the bar with a neutral grip and sit down, maintaining an erect posture by contracting your lower back. Your arms should be fully extended above you with your head straight and feet flat on the floor. Contract your lats to pull the bar down to your upper chest, bringing your elbows straight down. Squeeze your lats as you hold the peak contracted position for a brief count. Slowly return the handle along the same path and repeat.

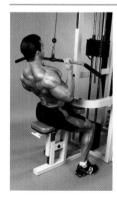

Reverse-Grip Pulldown

» Attach a long lat bar to the pulley and adjust the kneepad for a snug fit. Grasp the bar with a reverse, shoulder–width grip and sit down, maintaining erect posture by contracting your lower back. Your arms should be extended above you, your head straight and feet flat on the floor. Contract your lats to pull the bar to your upper chest, bringing your elbows straight down and behind you. Squeeze your shoulder blades together at the bottom and hold the peak contraction briefly. Slowly return the bar along the same path and repeat.

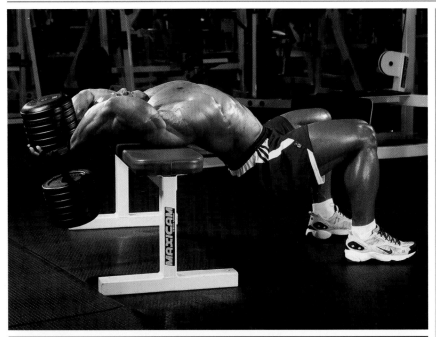

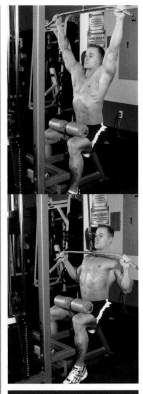

Pullover

» Lie perpendicular across a bench, with your upper back, head and neck supported by the bench. Your feet should be flat on the floor. Hold a dumbbell with your arms extended above your face. Keeping your arms straight, slowly lower the dumbbell back toward the top of your head, feeling a good stretch in your chest. Pause, then forcefully reverse direction with the dumbbell, squeezing your chest at the top.

Lat Pulldown

» Sit at a lat pulldown machine so the bar is directly overhead or slightly in front of your body. Adjust the pads so your quads fit snugly beneath. Grasp the angled ends of the bar with a wide, overhand grip. Keep your abs tight and back slightly arched with your feet flat on the floor. Squeeze your shoulder blades together and pull the bar down to your upper chest, keeping your elbows back and pointed out toward the sides in the same plane as your body. Squeeze and hold for a brief count before slowly allowing the bar up along the same path.

Standing Low Cable Row

» Stand facing the cable low pulley and grasp the V-bar. Bend your knees, keeping your back flat and chest up. Allow your arms to point directly toward the low pulley, fully extended. Keeping your abs tight, pull the handle into your lower abs. Squeeze your lats, then return to the start position.

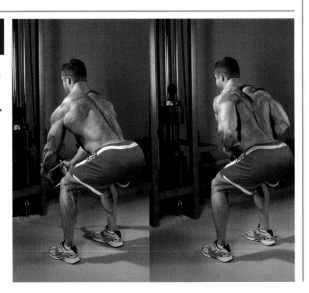

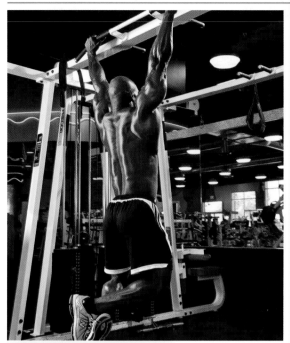

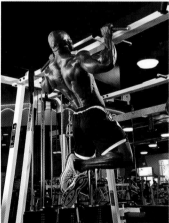

Pull-Up

» Grasp a fixed overhead bar with a wide overhand grip, your thumbs wrapped around the bar for safety. Hang freely from the bar, arms fully extended and feet crossed behind you. Contract your lats to raise your chin over the bar. Concentrate on keeping your elbows out to your sides, and pulling them down to your sides to raise yourself. Hold momentarily in the peak contracted position before lowering yourself down to the start.

Straight-Arm Kickback

» Bend over at the waist holding a dumbbell in one hand. Allow that arm to hang straight down toward the floor. Place your non-working hand on the same-side hip. Keeping your arm straight, kick your arm back until your entire arm reaches parallel with your torso. Squeeze your lat, then lower the dumbbell back to the start.

Rack Pull

» Inside a power rack, place the bar on the safeties just under knee level. Grasp the bar just outside your legs. Allow the bar to be flush against your legs. Keeping your abs tight, back flat, arms straight and chest up, press through the floor with your legs to raise the bar, dragging it up your quads until you are in a standing position. Lower the bar along the same path, allowing it to settle on the safety bars, then repeat.

Wide-Grip Seated Cable Row

» Sit at a row station and take a shoulder-width, palms-down grip on a straight-bar cable attachment. Bend your knees slightly and keep your back straight. Pull the bar all the way to your upper abs and squeeze your lats. Then slowly return the bar to the start, leaning forward just a bit to stretch your lats, but not so much that it causes you to round your lower back.

Dumbbell Deadlift

» Stand with your feet shoulder-width apart and a dumbbell outside each leg. Squat down and grasp the dumbbells, keeping your chest up and back flat. Press through the floor with your feet, extending at the knees and hips to pull the dumbbells upward until you're at a standing position. Squeeze your back, legs and glutes, then lower the dumbbells back to the floor.

CHEST

The mass-building workout included in the chart at right incorporates three variables that are crucial to adding size: 1) compound exercises in the form of barbell and dumbbell presses and dips; 2) high volume, as the workout consists of 17 total sets, including five each for the first two exercises; 3) rep ranges of 8–12 (the exception being two sets of six on the incline bench press), which is the optimal rep scheme for promoting hypertrophy. Weighted, not bodyweight, dips are included to maintain this rep range, since many individuals are able to exceed 12 reps without added resistance. The routine attacks all areas of the chest — upper, middle and lower pecs with incline presses, flat-bench dumbbell presses and decline flyes, respectively — to achieve overall development.

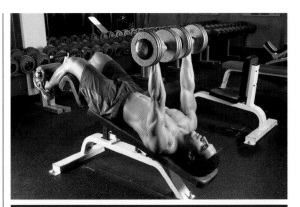

Decline Dumbbell Press

» Lie faceup on a decline bench set at about a 45-degree angle. Your torso should be fully supported from your head to your hips, with your knees bent and feet supported. Have a partner hand you a dumbbell in each hand. Extend your arms to hold the dumbbells up toward the ceiling with your palms forward. Bend your arms and slowly lower the dumbbells toward the outsides of your chest. (During the barbell version, the bar would come to your lower chest). When the dumbbells reach chest level, forcefully extend your arms, pressing the dumbbells back to the starting position.

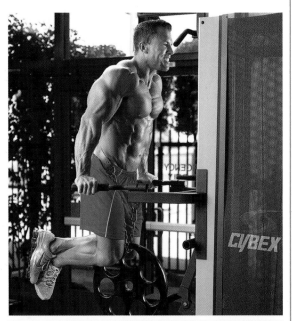

Weighted Dip

» With weight hanging around your waist, grasp the dip bars with your arms extended. Lean forward and bend your knees while keeping your legs crossed. Keep your elbows out to your sides as you bend them to lower your body down until your upper arms are about parallel to the floor. Press your hands into the bars to extend your arms and raise your body back up.

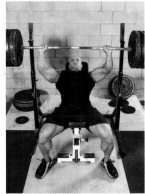

Incline Bench Press

» Lie on an incline bench set at approximately 30-45 degrees. Spread your legs with your feet flat on the floor. Grasp the barbell with a pronated (overhand) grip, wider than shoulder-width. Unrack the bar and hold it directly above your upper chest. Slowly lower the bar to your upper chest. Without bouncing the bar off of yourself, powerfully press it back up to the starting position. Pause momentarily in the top position before repeating for reps.

#11 LOWER CHEST PRIORITY

EXERCISE	SETS	REPS
Decline Bench Press	4	10, 10, 12, 12
Upright Cable Crossover	4	8, 8, 10, 10
Dumbbell Bench Press	3	10, 12, 15
Weighted Dip	3	to failure

#12 UPPER CHEST PRIORITY

EXERCISE	SETS	REPS
Incline Smith Press	4	6, 10, 12, 15
Incline Dumbbell Press	3	10, 10, 10
Incline Dumbbell Flye	3	8, 10, 12
Decline Push-Up	3	to failure

#13 MASS-BUILDING

EXERCISE	SETS	REPS
Incline Bench Press	5	6, 6, 8, 10, 12
Dumbbell Bench Press	5	8, 8, 10, 10, 12
Decline Dumbbell Flye	4	8, 8, 10, 12
Weighted Dip	3	8, 10, 12

#14 BEGINNER'S

EXERCISE	SETS	REPS
Machine Chest Press	4	10, 10, 12, 12
Machine Incline Press	3	10, 10, 10
Flat Dumbbell Flye	3	10, 10, 10

#15 AT-HOME

EXERCISE	SETS	REPS
Dumbbell Bench Press	4	8, 10, 12, 20
Incline Dumbbell Flye	4	10, 12, 12, 20
Decline Push-Up	4	to failure

#16 15-MINUTE WORKOUT

EXERCISE	SETS[1]	REPS
Smith Incline Press	3	6, 10, 15
Smith Bench Press	3	6, 10, 15
Smith Decline Press	3	6, 10, 15
Pec-Deck Flye	1	50

#17 GIANT-SET WORKOUT[2]

EXERCISE	SETS	REPS
Incline Dumbbell Flye	4	10, 10, 10, 10
Bench Press	4	10, 10, 10, 10
Decline Dumbbell Press	4	10, 10, 10, 10
Pec-Deck Flye	4	10, 10, 10, 10

#18 STRENGTH

EXERCISE	SETS[3]	REPS
Bench Press	4	4, 4, 6, 8
Incline Dumbbell Press	4	4, 4, 6, 8
Decline Bench Press	3	4, 6, 6
Flat Dumbbell Flye	3	4, 6, 6

#19 GET RIPPED

EXERCISE	SETS[1]	REPS
Incline Dumbbell Press	5	10, 12, 12, 15, 20
Flat Dumbbell Flye	4	12, 12, 15, 15
Pullover	4	15, 15, 20, 20
Weighted Dip	4	10, 12, 15, 20

#20 GET SUPER PUMPED

EXERCISE	SETS[1]	REPS
Smith Bench Press	4	10, 10, 30, 30
Flat Cable Flye	4	10, 10, 30, 30
Incline Cable Flye	4	10, 10, 30, 30

[1] Rest no more than 30 seconds between each set.
[2] A giant set consists of four or more exercises performed consecutively without rest as a means to increase intensity and promote muscle growth. Do one set of each exercise back-to-back — that's one giant set. Rest three minutes between each giant set.
[3] Rest 2–3 minutes between each set.
Notes: The above workouts don't include warm-up sets. Unless otherwise noted, rest 60–90 seconds between all sets.

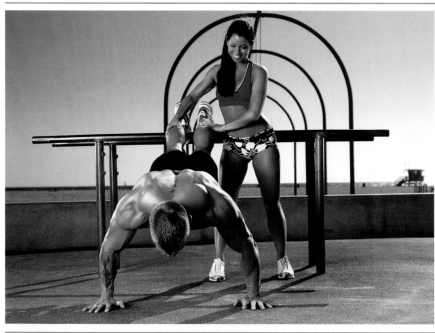

Decline Push-Up

» Place both of your feet on a bench or similar elevated surface, with your hands wider than shoulder-width and flat on the floor and your arms fully extended. Keeping your head neutral and abs tight, lower yourself toward the floor until your chest gently touches, then press through your hands until your arms are fully extended and repeat.

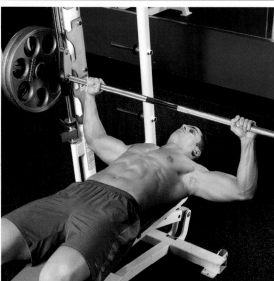

Smith Bench Press

» Place a bench centered inside a Smith machine. Grasp the bar with a wide, overhand grip. Rotate the bar to unrack it. Slowly lower the bar to your lower chest, pausing when the bar is just about an inch away from your pecs, then powerfully press the bar back up to full arm extension and repeat.

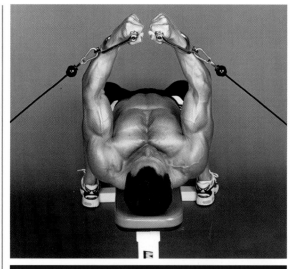

Flat Cable Flye

» Place a flat bench equidistant between two low pulley cables. Grasp the two D-handles attached to the cables and lie flat on the bench. Keeping your arms slightly bent, pull the handles in front of you, as if you were hugging a barrel, squeezing your chest when your hands are above your torso. Then lower the handles back to the start, stopping when your upper arms are parallel with the bench.

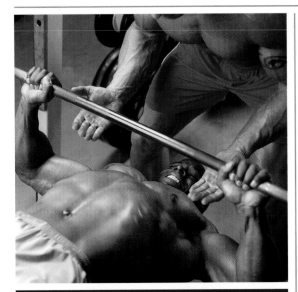

Decline Bench Press

» Lie face-up on a decline bench set at about a 45-degree angle. Your torso should be fully supported from your head to your hips, with your knees bent and feet supported, as well. Grasp the bar with a wide, overhand grip. Bend your arms and slowly lower the bar toward your lower chest. When the bar reaches chest level, forcefully extend your arms pressing the bar back to the starting position.

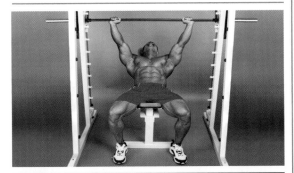

Smith Incline Press

» Lie on an incline bench set at approximately 30–45 degrees, placed inside a Smith machine. Spread your legs with your feet flat on the floor. Grasp the barbell with a pronated (overhand) grip, outside shoulder-width. Rotate and unrack the bar and hold it directly above your upper chest. Slowly lower the bar to your upper chest. Without bouncing the bar, power-fully press it back up to the starting position. Pause momentarily at the top before repeating for reps.

Smith Decline Press

» Lie face-up on a decline bench set at about a 45-degree angle, set inside a Smith machine. Your torso should be fully supported from your head to your hips, with your knees bent and feet tucked behind footrests. Grasp the bar with a wide, overhand grip and rotate the bar to unrack it and hold it directly above you. Bend your arms and slowly lower the bar toward your lower chest. When the bar reaches chest level, forcefully extend your arms, pressing the bar back to the starting position.

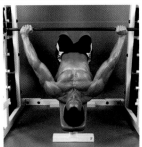

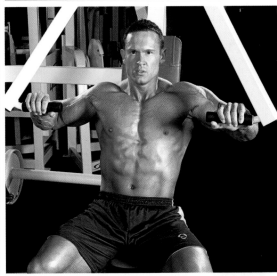

Incline Machine Press

» Adjust the machine so your back rests comfortably against the pad and your feet are flat on the floor. The handles should be aligned right at or just below shoulder level when you sit down. Press the handles away from you until your arms are fully extended without locking out your elbows. Slowly bring the handles back toward your chest without letting the weights touch the stack and repeat.

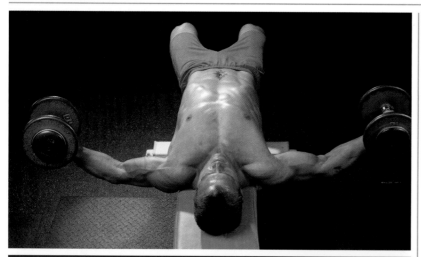

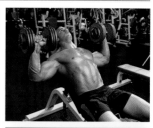

Incline Dumbbell Press

>> Adjust a bench so that the incline in the bench is 30–45 degrees. Lie face-up on the bench with your feet flat on the floor. Hold a dumbbell in each hand just outside your shoulders. Powerfully press the dumbbells upward toward the ceiling, stopping when the dumbbells are an inch or so away from each other, then slowly return the dumbbells to the start and repeat.

Flat Dumbbell Flye

>> Lie face-up on the bench with your feet flat on the floor. Hold a dumbbell in each hand with a neutral grip and extend your arms above your chest. Bend your elbows slightly. Slowly lower the dumbbells in a wide arc down to your sides. Keep your elbows locked in the slightly bent position throughout. Stop when your elbows reach shoulder level before reversing the motion.

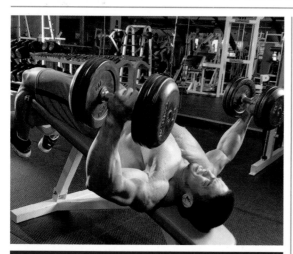

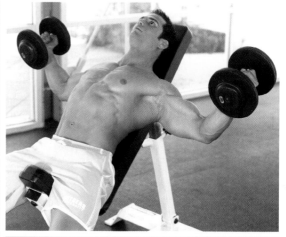

Decline Dumbbell Flye

>> Lie face-up on the decline bench with your feet secured under the pads. Hold a dumbbell in each hand with a neutral grip and extend your arms above your chest. Bend your elbows slightly. Slowly lower the dumbbells in a wide arc down to your sides. Keep your elbows locked in the slightly bent position throughout the range of motion. Stop when your elbows reach shoulder level before reversing the motion.

Incline Dumbbell Flye

>> Adjust a bench to roughly 30–45 degrees. Lie face-up with your feet flat on the floor. Hold a dumbbell in each hand with a neutral grip and extend your arms above your chest. Bend your elbows slightly. Slowly lower the dumbbells in a wide arc down to your sides. Keep your elbows locked in the slightly bent position throughout the range of motion. Stop when your elbows reach shoulder level before reversing the motion.

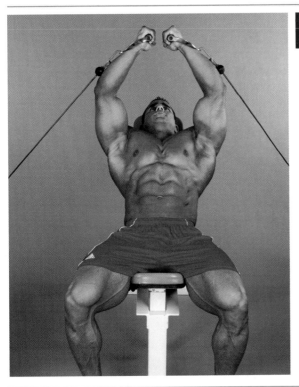

Incline Cable Flye

» Adjust a bench inside a cable crossover so that the incline in the bench is roughly 30–45 degrees. Lie face-up on the bench with your feet flat on the floor. Hold a D-handle in each hand with a neutral grip and extend your arms above your chest. Bend your elbows slightly. Slowly lower the handles in a wide arc out to your sides. Keep your elbows locked in the slightly bent position throughout the range of motion. Stop when your elbows reach shoulder level, then reverse the motion.

Upright Cable Crossover

» Attach D-handles to the upper pulleys on a cable-crossover machine. Stand in the direct center of the machine with your knees slightly bent, your focus forward. Grasp the handles with your palms facing down and bend your elbows slightly. Bring the handles down and below your waist close to your body, keeping your arms slightly bent. Pause a moment and squeeze the peak contraction before slowly allowing the handles to return to the start position.

Bench Press

» Lie face-up on a bench with your feet flat on the floor. Grasp the barbell with an overhand grip, your hands slightly wider than shoulder-width apart. Unrack the bar and slowly lower it toward your chest. Keep your wrists aligned with your elbows and your elbows pointed out to your sides. When the bar just touches your chest, press back up explosively, driving the weight away from you until your elbows are just short of locking out.

Dumbbell Bench Press

» Lie face-up on the bench with your feet flat on the floor. Hold a dumbbell in each hand just outside your shoulders. Powerfully press the dumbbells upward toward the ceiling, stopping when the dumbbells are an inch or so away from each other, then slowly return them to the start and repeat.

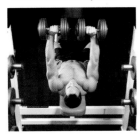

Pec-Deck Flye

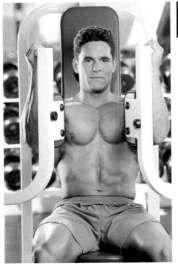

» Sit in the machine with your lower back fully supported and your feel flat on the floor. With your arms at 90-degree angles, place your lower arms flush against the pads and grasp the handles. Using your elbows, bring the handles together in front of your face, squeezing your chest hard, then slowly return to the start, stopping when your upper arms are perpendicular with your torso.

QUADS

Strong legs are often what make a decent body a complete one, and our quad strength workout will help you add size and power. It includes all the aspects any good strength routine needs: compound exercises that allow you to move a lot of weight; slightly lower volume (fewer total sets) than a typical mass-gaining workout so as not to exhaust your muscles too much; heavy weight with low reps (mostly 4–6); and, of course, longer rest periods to ensure adequate recovery between sets. The single-leg press is one exercise you don't often see in a hardcore strength routine, but it's great for determining whether one leg is weaker than the other and for promoting balanced strength in the lower body.

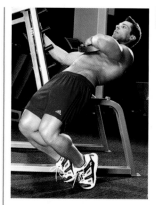

Sissy Squat

» Rise onto your toes, grasping a support for balance. Hold a weight plate across your chest with the other arm. Bend your knees and let them extend out in front of you, leaning back as you descend. At the bottom, simultaneously push through your toes and drive your hips forward and up.

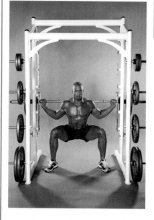

Wide-Stance Smith Squat

» Stand inside a Smith machine with the bar across your upper back, your legs spread wide and toes pointed outward. Keep your chest up, back flat. Rotate the bar to unrack it. Inhale, then bend your knees and hips to squat down as if sitting in a chair. Go as low as possible, then explode up to the start position.

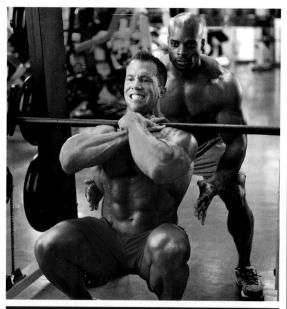

Smith Front Squat

» Stand inside a Smith machine with the bar across your front delts and upper chest. Cross your arms to build a shelf for the bar. Keep your chest up and back flat, eyes focused forward. With your abs tight, bend your knees and hips as if sitting in a chair until your thighs are well below parallel to the floor. Reverse motion by driving through your heels and pressing your hips forward to return to the start position.

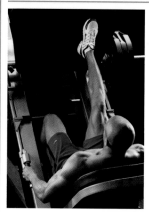

Single Leg Press

» Sit squarely in a leg press machine and place one foot on the sled. Keeping your chest up and lower back pressed into the back support, carefully unlock the weight from the safeties. Bend your knee to lower the weight. Hold for a brief count, then extend your leg to press the weight up. Stop just short of lockout, then repeat for the other leg. Or do all reps with one leg, then switch legs.

#21 MASS-BUILDING

EXERCISE	SETS	REPS
Squat	5	6, 6, 8, 10, 12
Leg Press	5	8, 8, 10, 10, 12
Hack Squat	4	8, 8, 10, 12
Leg Extension	3	8, 10, 12

#22 BEGINNER'S

EXERCISE	SETS	REPS
Smith Squat	4	10, 10, 12, 12
Leg Press	3	10, 10, 10
Lunge	3	10, 10, 10
Leg Extension	3	10, 10, 10

#23 AT-HOME

EXERCISE	SETS	REPS
Dumbbell Squat	4	8, 10, 12, 20
Sissy Squat	4	10, 12, 12, 20
Dumbbell Step-Up	4	12, 12, 15, 20

#24 15-MINUTE WORKOUT

EXERCISE	SETS[1]	REPS
Leg Extension	3	6, 10, 15
Machine Leg Press	3	6, 10, 15
Bodyweight Jump Squat	3	to failure

#25 INNER QUAD PRIORITY

EXERCISE	SETS	REPS
Wide-Stance Smith Squat	4	10, 10, 12, 12
High and Wide Leg Press	4	8, 8, 10, 10
Leg Extension (toes out)	4	10, 12, 15, 15

#26 OUTER QUAD PRIORITY

EXERCISE	SETS	REPS
Narrow-Stance Hack Squat	4	6, 10, 12, 15
Smith Front Squat	3	10, 10, 10
Sissy Squat	3	8, 10, 12
Leg Extension (toes in)	3	8, 10, 12

#27 GIANT-SET WORKOUT[2]

EXERCISE	SETS	REPS
Leg Extension	4	10, 10, 10, 10
Hack Squat	4	10, 10, 10, 10
Leg Press	4	10, 10, 10, 10
Smith Front Squat	4	10, 10, 10, 10

#28 STRENGTH

EXERCISE	SETS[3]	REPS
Squat	4	4, 4, 6, 8
Single-Leg Press	4	4, 4, 6, 8
Hack Squat	3	4, 6, 6

#29 GET RIPPED

EXERCISE	SETS[1]	REPS
Leg Extension	5	10, 12, 12, 15, 20
Leg Press	4	12, 12, 15, 15
Smith Front Squat	4	15, 15, 20, 20
Sissy Squat	4	10, 12, 15, 20

#30 GET SUPER PUMPED

EXERCISE	SETS[1]	REPS
Squat	4	10, 10, 30, 30
Leg Press	4	10, 10, 30, 30
Leg Extension	4	10, 10, 30, 30

1 Rest no more than 30 seconds between each set.
2 A giant set consists of four or more exercises performed consecutively without rest as a means to increase intensity and promote muscle growth. Do one set of each exercise back-to-back — that's one giant set. Rest three minutes between each giant set.
3 Rest 2–3 minutes between each set.
Notes: The above workouts don't include warm-up sets. Unless otherwise noted, rest 60–90 seconds between all sets.

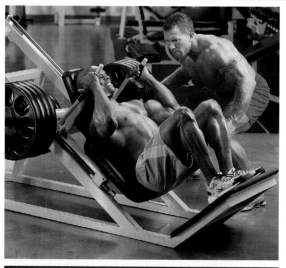

Smith Squat

>> Stand inside a Smith machine with the bar across your upper back and your feet just outside shoulder width, toes pointed out slightly. Keep your chest up and back flat, eyes focused forward. With your abs tight, bend your knees and hips as if sitting in a chair until your thighs are parallel with the floor. Reverse motion by driving through your heels and pressing your hips forward to return to the start position.

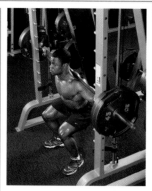

Hack Squat

>> Step inside a hack squat machine, placing your shoulders and back against the pads. Your feet should be fairly close together and low on the platform; keep your feet flat throughout the exercise. Maintain good posture, with your chest up and abs pulled in tight. Unhook the safety bars, and slowly lower yourself into the bottom position, stopping when your legs are well beyond parallel to the ground. Pause then forcefully press yourself upward to the start position, keeping your knees bent slightly. Squeeze your legs and begin the next repetition.

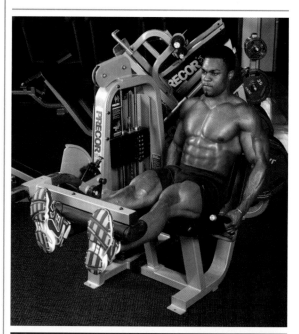

Squat

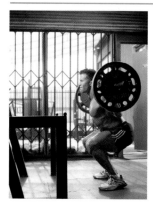

>> Stand erect holding a bar across your upper back with your feet about shoulder–width apart, knees slightly bent and your toes turned out. Keeping your head neutral, abs tight and torso erect, bend at the knees and hips to slowly lower your body, as if you were going to sit down in a chair. Pause when your legs reach a 90–degree angle, then forcefully drive through your heels, extending at your hips and knees until you arrive at the standing position.

Leg Extension

>> Adjust the seat for your body frame, then sit squarely in the machine. Hook your feet under the padded bar. Keep you head straight and hold the handles for stability. With your feet pointed forward, extend your legs out as high as you can, while remaining seated flat on the machine. Squeeze your quads hard at the top, then slowly lower the weight until just short of the weight stack touching.

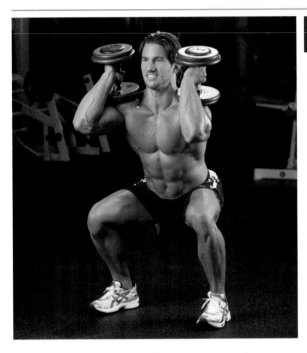

Dumbbell Squat

» Stand erect holding dumbbells atop your shoulders or hanging at your sides, with your feet wider than shoulder-width apart, knees slightly bent and your toes turned out slightly. Keeping your head neutral, abs tight and torso erect, bend at the knees and hips to slowly lower your body, as if you were going to sit down in a chair. Pause when your legs reach a 90-degree angle, then forcefully drive through your heels, extending at your hips and knees until you arrive at the standing position.

Dumbbell Step-Up

» Place a knee-high step in front of you and grasp a dumbbell in each hand. Stand with your feet in a comfortable shoulder-width stance. Step forward with one leg onto the step and drive through that thigh to lift your body upward. Bring the trailing leg to the top of the step and stand on the box, then step back with the opposite leg to the floor and lower yourself. Repeat, then switch legs.

High-and-Wide Leg Press

» Place your feet on the sled, high and wide, toes pointed out. Bend your knees to lower the weight, stopping before your glutes lift off the pad. Hold for a brief count, then extend your legs to press the weight up, stopping just short of locking out your legs, and repeat.

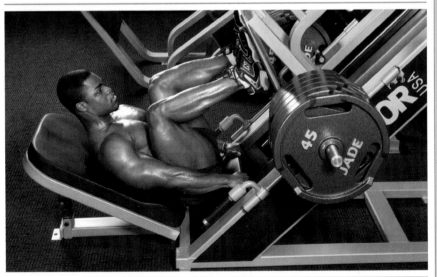

Leg Press

» Sit squarely in the leg press machine and place your feet on the sled, shoulder-width apart. Keeping your chest up and lower back pressed into the back support, carefully unlock the weight from the safeties. Bend your knees to lower the weight, stopping before your glutes lift off the pad. Hold for a brief count, then extend your legs to press the weight up, stopping just short of locking out your knees. Squeeze your legs hard at the top, then repeat for reps.

NOTE: For bodyweight jump squat, see page 31.

HAMSTRINGS/GLUTES

The hamstrings are one of the toughest muscle groups to train at home, since most of us rely on leg curl machines at the gym to train the backs of our thighs. That said, the at-home hammie routine provides an intense training session to help you build bigger legs. An important caveat concerns exercises such as squats, leg presses and lunges, which mainly work the quads but will also stress the hams and glutes if performed through a full range of motion. There's a lot of crossover in the routines featured at right; complete isolation of just the hamstrings often isn't possible or even necessary. Your hammies will still get a great workout, even if your quads and glutes come into play a bit.

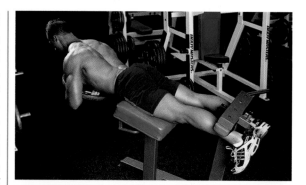

Weighted Glute-Ham Raise

» On a back extension bench, secure your ankles under the pads. Hold a plate across your chest. Your torso and thighs should be straight while your lower legs are at a 90–degree angle to the thighs. Slowly extend your legs by lowering your torso and thighs together toward the floor. Flex your hams to bring your body back to vertical.

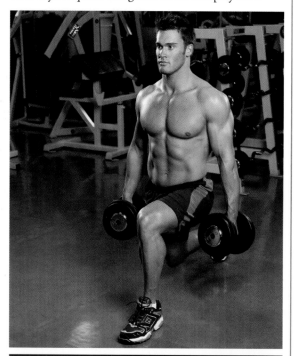

Dumbbell Lunge

» Holding dumbbells in each hand, step forward with one foot. Bend both knees to lower yourself, making sure your front knee doesn't pass your toes. Stop just short of your rear knee touching the floor and reverse directions, driving through the heel of your forward foot to return to the start.

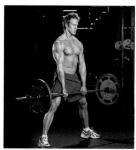

Sumo Deadlift

» Take a wide stance and place your shins against the bar, toes out slightly. Let your arms hang straight down, forearms on the inside of your thighs. Grab the bar with an alternated grip. Dip your hips a bit, then start your pull, pressing through the floor with your feet and dragging the bar up your legs. Push through your heels as you stand up with the bar, then lower along the same path.

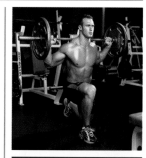

Barbell Lunge

» Holding a barbell across your upper back, step forward with one foot. Bend both knees to lower yourself, making sure your front knee doesn't pass your toes. Stop just short of your rear knee touching the floor and reverse directions, driving through the heel of your forward foot to return to the start.

#31 MASS-BUILDING

EXERCISE	SETS	REPS
Squat	5	6, 6, 8, 10, 12
Romanian Deadlift	5	8, 8, 10, 10, 12
Good Morning	4	8, 8, 10, 12
Leg Curl	3	8, 10, 12

#32 BEGINNER'S

EXERCISE	SETS	REPS
Leg Press	4	10, 10, 12, 12
Leg Curl	3	10, 10, 10
Dumbbell Lunge	3	10, 10, 10

#33 AT-HOME

EXERCISE	SETS	REPS
Reverse Hamstring Curl	4	30-second hold
Exercise Ball Roll-In	4	10, 12, 12, 20
Dumbbell Romanian Deadlift	4	12, 12, 15, 20

#34 15-MINUTE WORKOUT

EXERCISE	SETS[1]	REPS
Smith Romanian Deadlift	3	6, 10, 15
Reverse Hamstring Extension	3	6, 10, 15
Weighted Glute-Ham Raise	3	6, 10, 15

#35 INNER HAMSTRING PRIORITY

EXERCISE	SETS	REPS
Sumo Deadlift	4	10, 10, 12, 12
Seated Leg Curl (toes in)	4	8, 8, 10, 10
Lunge	4	10, 12, 14, 15

#36 OUTER HAMSTRING PRIORITY

EXERCISE	SETS	REPS
Squat	4	6, 10, 12, 15
Stiff-Legged Deadlift	3	10, 10, 10
Lying Leg Curl (toes out)	3	8, 10, 12
Barbell Step-Up	3	8, 10, 12

#37 GIANT-SET WORKOUT[2]

EXERCISE	SETS	REPS
Smith Squat	4	10, 10, 10, 10
Lying Leg Curl	4	10, 10, 10, 10
Weighted Glute-Ham Raise	4	10, 10, 10, 10
Dumbbell Romanian Deadlift	4	10, 10, 10, 10

#38 STRENGTH

EXERCISE	SETS[3]	REPS
Barbell Hack Squat	4	4, 4, 6, 8
Romanian Deadlift	4	4, 4, 6, 8
Good Morning	4	4, 4, 6, 8

#39 GET RIPPED

EXERCISE	SETS[1]	REPS
Leg Press	5	10, 12, 12, 15, 20
Dumbbell Deadlift	4	12, 12, 15, 15
Leg Curl	4	15, 15, 20, 20
Split Jump Squat	4	to failure

#40 GET SUPER PUMPED

EXERCISE	SETS[1]	REPS
Squat	4	10, 10, 30, 30
Romanian Deadlift	4	10, 10, 30, 30
Weighted Glute-Ham Raise	4	10, 10, 30, 30

1 Rest no more than 30 seconds between each set.
2 A giant set consists of four or more exercises performed consecutively without rest as a means to increase intensity and promote muscle growth. Do one set of each exercise back-to-back — that's one giant set. Rest three minutes between each giant set.
3 Rest 2–3 minutes between each set.
Notes: The above workouts don't include warm-up sets. Unless otherwise noted, rest 60–90 seconds between all sets.

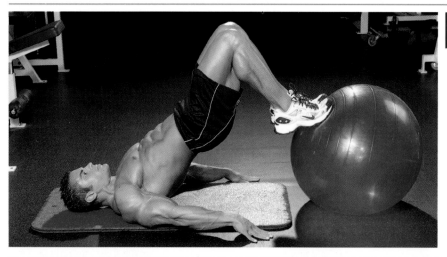

Exercise Ball Roll-In

» Lie on the floor with your calves on top of an exercise ball. With your arms flat on the floor, raise your body to form a bridge from feet to shoulders. Flex your hamstrings to curl the ball toward your glutes. Squeeze your hams and glutes, then roll the ball back to the start and repeat.

Barbell Hack Squat

» Stand in front of a barbell loaded with the appropriate weight with your feet shoulder-width apart. Bend slightly at the hips and, keeping your back flat and chest out, bend your knees to grasp the bar with a shoulder-width, palms-down grip just outside your feet. Maintaining good posture, contract your quads and glutes and then, with an explosive movement, stand up until your knees are just short of locked out.

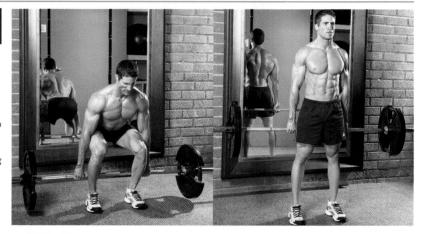

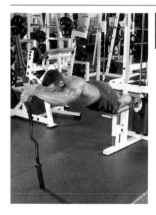

Reverse Ham Curl

» Kneel reversed on a lat pulldown station, securing your ankles under the pads. Hold an empty barbell in front of you. Keeping your body (from knees to shoulders) straight, lower yourself, flexing your hams until your body reaches the floor. With the empty barbell as a self-spot, pull with your hamstrings to raise yourself upright to the start position.

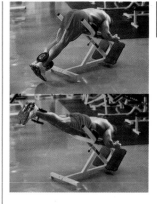

Reverse Ham Extension

» Adjust the upper pad of a back extension bench; bend at the waist. Lean over the bench and grasp the footpads for stability, allowing your legs to angle toward the floor. With a dumbbell between your ankles and a flat back, raise your legs till your body forms a straight line. Squeeze your hamstrings, glutes and low back. Lower and repeat.

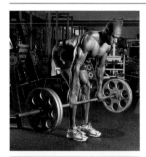

Romanian Deadlift

» Stand upright holding a barbell in front of your upper thighs with a pronated (overhand) grip. Keep your feet shoulder–width apart and a slight bend in your knees. Keeping your chest up, abs tight and the natural arch in your low back, lean forward from your hips, pushing them rearward until your torso is roughly parallel to the floor. As you lean forward, keep your arms straight and slide the bar down your thighs toward the floor until it reaches your shins. At the bottom, keep your back flat, head neutral with the bar very close to your legs. Flex your hamstrings and glutes and lift your torso while pushing your hips forward until you bring the bar back to the start position.

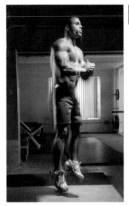

Jump Squat

» Stand with both hands directly in front of you, knees slightly bent with roughly a shoulder–width stance. Keeping your chest up and back flat, squat down until your thighs approach parallel with the floor, then explode upward as high as possible, allowing your feet to leave the floor. Land on soft feet with your knees bent and repeat immediately.

Dumbbell Step-Up

» Place a knee–high step in front of you and grasp a dumbbell in each hand. Stand with your feet in a comfortable shoulder–width stance. Place one leg on the step and drive through that thigh to bring your body upward. Bring the trailing leg up so you're standing on the step. Lower yourself with the opposite leg. Repeat, then switch legs.

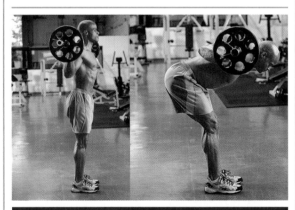

Good Morning

» Set a barbell across your upper back. Set your feet at shoulder–width and bend slightly at your knees. With your torso high and eyes straight ahead, start the movement by pushing your glutes back and bending forward at the waist. Descend forward until your torso is parallel to the floor. Pause deliberately at the bottom before contracting your lower back, glutes and hamstrings to raise your torso back to the starting position.

Leg Curl

» Lie face-down on a leg-curl machine and position your Achilles' tendons below the padded lever, your knees just off the edge of the bench. Grasp the bench or handles for stability. Bend your knees slightly to protect them from overextension. Raise your feet toward your glutes in a strong, deliberate motion. Squeeze at the top, then lower to the start position.

Smith Romanian Deadlift

» Place the bar of a Smith at thigh level. Stand erect, knees soft, feet hip-width apart. Hold a slight arch in the lower back, with the bar close to your thighs. Grasp the bar just outside your hips. Lean forward, pushing your hips rearward as the bar slides toward midshin level and your upper body approaches parallel with the floor. Stop before your low back rounds. Maintain the arch as you rise back up, pushing your hips forward.

Split Jump Squat

» Step forward with one leg, as in a lunge. Keeping your chest up and back flat, bend both legs, lowering yourself toward the floor, then explode upward as high as possible, switching front and back legs in the air. Land on soft feet with your knees bent and repeat immediately.

SHOULDERS/TRAPS

Training a relatively small bodypart (abs, calves, forearms) in 15 minutes is no big deal, but getting a sufficient shoulder workout in that time is a much bigger challenge. The 15-minute workout at right, however, makes it possible with only nine total sets and 30-second rest periods. Most important, all three exercises use the same equipment (dumbbells and a low-back seat), so no relocation is necessary. Being short on time doesn't mean you have to shortchange your shoulder development. All three heads get attention — front and middle delts with overhead presses, middle delts with lateral raises and rear delts with bent-over laterals.

#41 MASS-BUILDING

EXERCISE	SETS	REPS
Overhead Press	5	6, 6, 8, 10, 12
Upright Row	5	8, 8, 10, 10, 12
Lateral Raise	4	8, 8, 10, 12
Bent-Over Lateral Raise	3	8, 10, 12

#42 BEGINNER'S

EXERCISE	SETS	REPS
Machine Overhead Press	4	10, 10, 12, 12
Cable Lateral Raise	3	10, 10, 10
Barbell Front Raise	3	10, 10, 10
Reverse Pec-Deck Flye	3	10, 10, 10

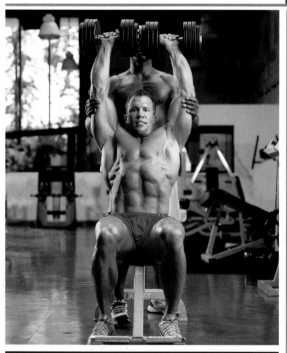

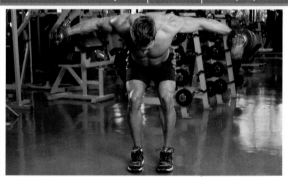

Bent-Over Lateral Raise

» With a dumbbell in each hand, chest up, back flat and knees soft, bend over at the waist until your torso is about parallel to the floor. Let the dumbbells hang directly beneath you. Keeping your arms slightly bent, powerfully raise the dumbbells up and out to your sides until your upper arms are about parallel with your torso. Slowly lower the dumbbells back to the start position and repeat.

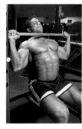

Overhead Press

» Sit against the back pad, lower back slightly arched and feet flat on the floor. Grasp the bar beyond shoulder width, palms forward, elbows pointing down and outward. Unrack the bar and hold it at shoulder level. In a smooth, strong motion, press straight up to just short of elbow lockout. Squeeze, lower the bar under control to the start and repeat for reps.

Overhead Dumbbell Press

» Sit on a low back bench, holding a dumbbell in each hand above shoulder level with a pronated grip (palms facing forward). Keep your head straight, eyes focused forward, and your shoulders back. Press the dumbbells overhead in an arc, but don't let the weights touch at the top. Slowly lower to the start position and repeat.

#43 AT-HOME

EXERCISE	SETS	REPS
Arnold Press	4	8, 10, 12, 20
Seated Lateral Raise	4	10, 12, 12, 20
Dumbbell Upright Row	4	12, 12, 15, 20
Seated Bent-Over Lateral Raise	3	12, 15, 15

#44 15-MINUTE WORKOUT

EXERCISE	SETS[1]	REPS
Seated Overhead Dumbbell Press	3	6, 10, 15
Seated Lateral Raise	3	6, 10, 15
Seated Bent-Over Lateral Raise	3	6, 10, 15

#45 FRONT DELT PRIORITY

EXERCISE	SETS	REPS
Upright Row	4	10, 10, 12, 12
90-Degree Arnold Press	4	8, 8, 10, 10
Barbell Front Raise	3	10, 12, 15
Reverse Pec-Deck Flye	3	10, 12, 15

#46 MIDDLE DELT PRIORITY & TRAPS

EXERCISE	SETS	REPS
Behind-the-Neck Press	4	6, 10, 12, 15
Lateral Raise	3	10, 10, 10
Smith Upright Row	3	8, 10, 12
Bent-Over Cable Lateral Raise	3	8, 10, 12
Barbell Shrug	3	8, 10, 12

#47 GIANT-SET WORKOUT[2]

EXERCISE	SETS	REPS
Overhead Dumbbell Press	4	10, 10, 10, 10
Seated Lateral Raise	4	10, 10, 10, 10
Dumbbell Front Raise	4	10, 10, 10, 10
Bent-Over Lateral Raise	4	10, 10, 10, 10

#48 STRENGTH

EXERCISE	SETS[3]	REPS
Overhead Press	4	4, 4, 6, 8
Upright Row	4	4, 4, 6, 8
Cable Lateral Raise	3	4, 6, 6
Reverse Pec-Deck Flye	3	4, 6, 6

#49 GET RIPPED

EXERCISE	SETS[1]	REPS
Smith Upright Row	5	10, 12, 12, 15, 20
Cable Front Raise	4	12, 12, 15, 15
Cable Lateral Raise	4	15, 15, 20, 20
Dumbbell Shrug	4	10, 12, 15, 20

#50 GET SUPER PUMPED

EXERCISE	SETS[1]	REPS
Overhead Dumbbell Press	4	10, 10, 30, 30
Dumbbell Upright Row	4	10, 10, 30, 30
Reverse Pec-Deck Flye	4	10, 10, 30, 30

1 Rest no more than 30 seconds between each set.
2 A giant set consists of four or more exercises performed consecutively without rest as a means to increase intensity and promote muscle growth. Do one set of each exercise back-to-back — that's one giant set. Rest three minutes between each giant set.
3 Rest 2–3 minutes between each set.
Notes: The above workouts don't include warm-up sets.
Unless otherwise noted, rest 60–90 seconds between all sets.

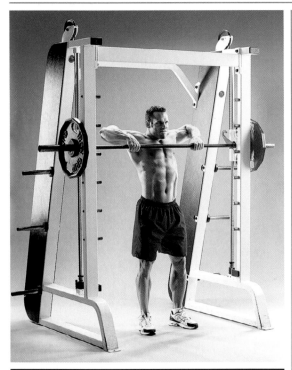

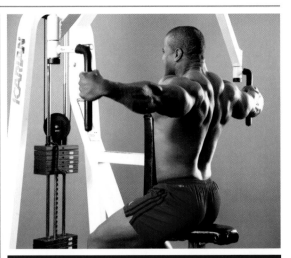

Reverse Pec-Deck Flye

» Sit reversed at a pec deck, and grasp the handles in front of you with a neutral grip. Keep your abs tight and your chest up. Flex your rear delts, keeping a slight bend in your elbows to pull the handles back until your upper arms are just passed perpendicular to your torso. Hold briefly, then return to the start.

Smith Upright Row

» inside a Smith machine with your feet shoulder-width apart, stand erect holding the bar in front of your thighs with a wide, pronated (overhand) grip. Maintain a slight bend in your knees. Keep your head straight and abs tight. Rotate the bar to unrack it. Flex your shoulders and pull the bar straight up toward your chin, bringing your elbows high. Keep the bar close to your body during the entire movement. In the top position, your elbows will be high and pointing out to your sides. Hold for a second before slowly lowering to the start position.

Dumbbell Shrug

» Stand holding a dumbbell in each hand at your sides. Keeping your chest up and abs tight, shrug your shoulders straight up toward the ceiling, squeezing your traps at the top. Slowly reverse the motion to lower back to the start.

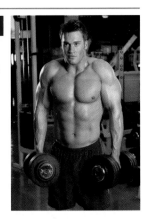

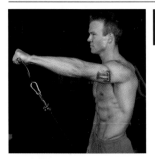

Cable Front Raise

» Stand facing away from a low cable pulley, holding a D-handle in one hand. Keeping your arm straight, raise the cable to just above parallel. Squeeze your shoulder, then slowly lower to the start.

Barbell Shrug

» Stand holding a barbell directly in front of your quads. Keeping your chest up and abs tight, shrug your shoulders straight up toward the ceiling, squeezing your traps at the top. Slowly reverse the motion to lower back to the start.

Lateral Raise

» Stand with your feet shoulder-width apart. Keep your abs tight, chest up and shoulders back. With your head straight, hold the dumbbells at your sides with a neutral grip. Without using momentum, raise the dumbbells out to your sides in a wide arc, keeping your elbows and hands moving together in the same plane. Raise the dumbbells just above shoulder level and hold momentarily in the peak contracted position. Slowly lower the dumbbells down along the same path and repeat for reps.

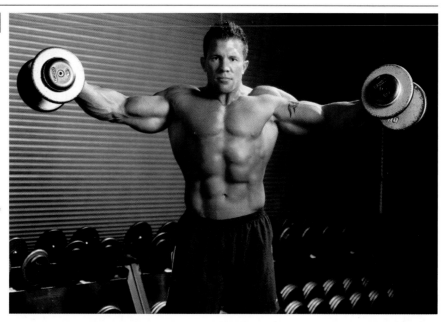

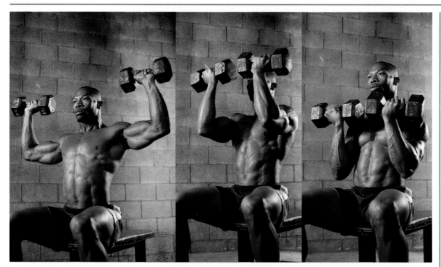

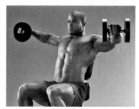

Seated Lateral Raise

» Sit on a low-back bench with your feet flat on the floor. With your head straight, hold the dumbbells at your sides with a neutral grip. This is your starting position. Without using momentum, raise the dumbbells out to your sides in a wide arc, elbows and hands moving together in the same plane. Raise the dumbbells to shoulder level and hold the peak contraction momentarily. Slowly lower the weights along the same path and repeat for reps.

90-Degree Arnold Press

» Sit in a low-back bench and hold a dumbbell in each hand above shoulder level with a pronated grip (palms facing forward), your head straight and eyes focused forward. Keeping your shoulders back, press the dumbbells overhead in an arc, but don't let the weights touch at the top. Slowly lower to the start position. When the dumbbells reach the start position, rotate your arms in front of your body, keeping your elbows high the entire time. Rotate the dumbbells until they are directly in front of your eyes and your palms face back toward you. Hold briefly, then rotate your arms outward until you reach the start of the dumbbell press position, press them upward and repeat.

Upright Row

» With your feet shoulder-width apart, stand erect holding a barbell in front of your thighs with a wide, pronated (overhand) grip. Maintain a slight bend in your knees. Keep your head straight and abs tight. This is your starting position. Flex your shoulders and pull the barbell straight up toward your chin, bringing your elbows high. The bar should be close to your body during the entire movement. Keep your torso erect and the natural curve in your spine throughout the exercise. In the top position, your elbows will be high and pointing out to your sides. Hold for a second before slowly lowering to the start position.

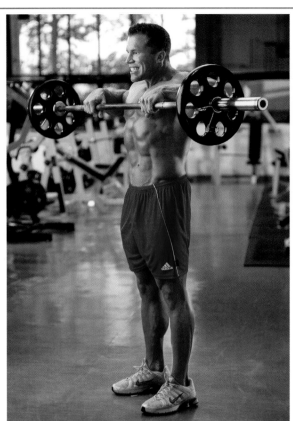

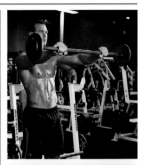

Barbell Front Raise

» Stand holding a loaded barbell directly in front of your thighs, your abs tight and chest up. Keeping your arms straight, raise the barbell in front of you just above parallel to the floor. Pause, then lower to the start and repeat.

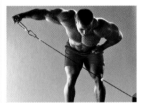

Bent-Over Cable Lateral Raise

» Stand sideways to a low cable pulley and grasp a D-handle, non-working hand on your hip for balance. With your chest up and knees soft, bend at the waist until your torso is about parallel to the floor. Let the working arm hang beneath you. Keeping your arm slightly bent, raise the handle up and out until your upper arm is parallel with your torso. Squeeze, then lower your arm back to the start and repeat.

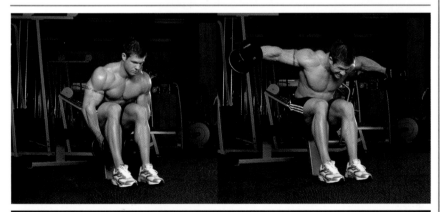

Seated Bent-Over Lateral Raise

» Sit at the end of a bench with a dumbbell in each hand. Bend over at the waist keeping your chest up, allowing the dumbbells to hang straight down and underneath your legs. Remaining in the bent-over position with a slight bend in your arms, raise the dumbbells up and out to your sides, squeezing your rear delts at the top. Slowly lower to the start and repeat.

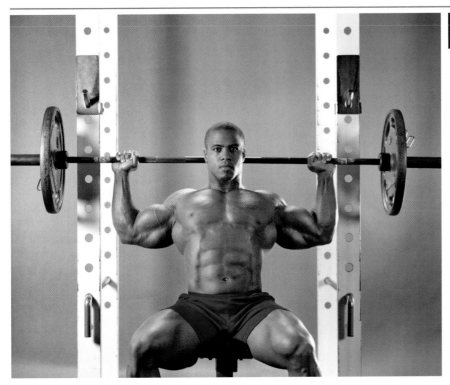

Behind-the-Neck Press

» Sit erect against the back pad support at the overhead press station or power rack. Keep your low back slightly arched and your feet flat on the floor. Grasp the bar with a wide, outside of shoulder width, palms–forward grip, elbows pointing down and outward. Carefully unrack the bar and hold it at shoulder level. In a smooth, strong motion, press the bar straight up to just short of elbow lockout. Squeeze, then lower the bar under control behind your head until the bar reaches the middle of the back of your head. Pause, then press the bar straight over your head and repeat.

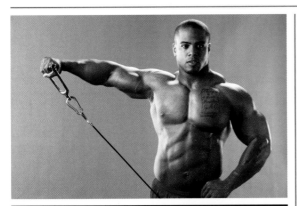

Cable Lateral Raise

» Stand sideways to a low cable pulley, feet shoulder-width apart, abs tight, chest up and shoulders back. With your head straight, grasp a D-handle with your hand opposite the machine. Without using momentum, raise the cable out to your sides in a wide arc, keeping your elbow and hand moving together in the same plane. Bring the cable just above shoulder level and hold the peak contraction briefly. Slowly lower the cable along the same path and repeat for reps.

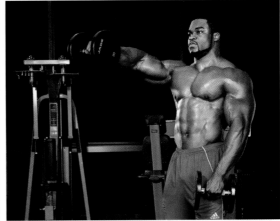

Dumbbell Front Raise

» Stand holding dumbbells in each hand in front of your thighs, your abs tight and chest up. Keeping your arms straight, raise one dumbbell in front of you just above parallel to the floor. Pause, then lower to the start and repeat with the other arm.

BICEPS

The biceps muscles provide arguably the most satisfying pump, so that at the end of an intense workout the sleeves of your T-shirt will feel as if they're two sizes too small. The "Get Super Pumped" workout at right was designed to stretch your sleeves just a bit more to help spark long-term muscle growth and assist you in breaking through even the most stubborn plateau. Exercise selection is fairly basic, with the only possible exception being the high-cable curl, chosen for the constant tension cables provide. The hallmark of the routine is the high-rep sets (30 reps), which increase blood flow to the working muscles, preceded by sets of 10 reps to promote hypertrophy.

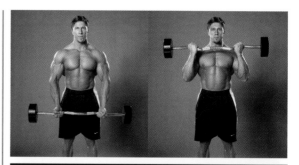

EZ-Bar Curl

» Stand holding an EZ bar with a shoulder–width grip, arms extended. Keep your abs tight, chest up and head straight. Contract your biceps to curl the bar toward your chest, keeping your elbows at your sides. Hold and squeeze at the top, then slowly return the bar along the same path. Repeat for reps.

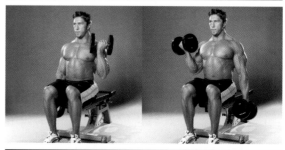

Seated Alternating Dumbbell Curl

» Sit on a low back bench, holding a dumbbell in each hand at your sides. Keeping your chest up, curl one dumbbell up toward the same-side shoulder, squeezing your biceps hard at the top, then lower to the start. Repeat with the other arm.

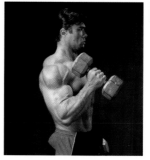

Hammer Curl

» Stand holding a dumbbell in each hand with a neutral grip. Curl one arm at a time, maintaining the palms–in grip. Squeeze your biceps and forearm at the top of each rep and return to the start. Repeat with the opposite arm.

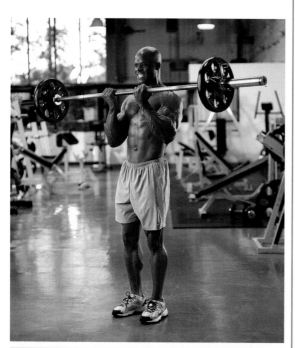

Close-Grip Barbell Curl

» Stand holding a barbell with a narrow, underhand grip, arms extended, your abs tight, chest up and head straight. Contract your biceps to curl the bar toward your chest, keeping your elbows at your sides. Hold and squeeze at the top, then slowly return the bar along the same path. Repeat for reps.

#51 MASS-BUILDING

EXERCISE	SETS	REPS
Barbell Curl	4	6, 8, 10, 12
Preacher Curl	4	6, 8, 10, 12
Incline Dumbbell Curl	4	8, 8, 10, 12
High-Cable Curl	3	8, 10, 12

#52 BEGINNER'S

EXERCISE	SETS	REPS
EZ-Bar Curl	4	10, 10, 12, 12
Machine Preacher Curl	3	10, 10, 10
Cable Concentration Curl	3	10, 10, 10

#53 AT-HOME

EXERCISE	SETS	REPS
Dumbbell Curl	4	10, 12, 12, 20
Dumbbell Curl (21s)[1]	4	21
Concentration Curl	4	12, 12, 15, 20

#54 15-MINUTE WORKOUT

EXERCISE	SETS[2]	REPS
Cable Curl	3	6, 10, 15
High-Cable Curl	3	6, 10, 15
Cable Concentration Curl	3	6, 10, 15

#55 BICEPS OUTER HEAD ("PEAK") PRIORITY

EXERCISE	SETS	REPS
Close-Grip Barbell Curl	4	10, 10, 12, 12
Incline Dumbbell Curl	4	8, 8, 10, 10
Hammer Curl	4	10, 12, 15, 15
Cable Curl	3	10, 10, 12

#56 BICEPS SHORT HEAD PRIORITY

EXERCISE	SETS	REPS
Dumbbell Preacher Curl	4	6, 10, 12, 15
Scott Curl	3	10, 10, 10
Dumbbell Curl	3	8, 10, 12
Wide-Grip Barbell Curl	3	8, 10, 12

#57 GIANT-SET WORKOUT[3]

EXERCISE	SETS	REPS
Preacher Curl	4	10, 10, 10, 10
Scott Curl	4	10, 10, 10, 10
Incline Dumbbell Curl	4	10, 10, 10, 10
Dumbbell Curl	4	10, 10, 10, 10

#58 STRENGTH

EXERCISE	SETS[4]	REPS
Barbell Curl	4	4, 4, 6, 8
Smith Machine Drag Curl	4	4, 4, 6, 8
Hammer Curl	4	4, 4, 6, 8

#59 GET RIPPED

EXERCISE	SETS[2]	REPS
Alternating Dumbbell Curl	5	10, 12, 12, 15, 20
Preacher Curl	4	12, 12, 15, 15
Dumbbell Curl (21s)[1]	4	21

#60 GET SUPER PUMPED

EXERCISE	SETS[2]	REPS
Barbell Curl	4	10, 10, 30, 30
High-Cable Curl	4	10, 10, 30, 30
Hammer Curl	4	10, 10, 30, 30

[1] For each set, do seven reps using just the bottom half of the range of motion, followed by seven reps using just the top half of the range of motion, followed by seven reps using a full range of motion.
[2] Rest no more than 30 seconds between each set.
[3] A giant set consists of four or more exercises performed consecutively without rest as a means to increase intensity and promote muscle growth. Do one set of each exercise back-to-back — that's one giant set. Rest three minutes between each giant set.
[4] Rest 2–3 minutes between each set.
Note: The above workouts don't include warm-up sets. Unless otherwise noted, rest 60–90 seconds between all sets.

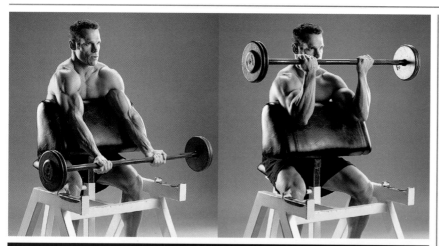

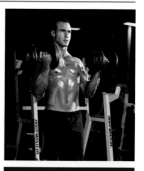

Dumbbell Curl

>> Stand holding a pair of dumbbells at your sides, arms extended. Keep your abs tight, chest up and head straight. Contract your biceps to curl the dumbbells toward your shoulders, keeping your elbows at your sides. Hold and squeeze at the top, then slowly return the dumbbells along the same path.

Preacher Curl

>> Set up a preacher bench so that the top of the pad fits securely under your armpits. Take a shoulder–width, underhand grip on the bar and position your arms parallel to each other on the bench. Keep your feet flat on the floor and your head straight. This is your starting position. Flex your biceps to bring the bar as high as possible without allowing your elbows to flare out. Squeeze your biceps hard at the top before slowly returning the bar to the starting position. Stop just short of full-arm extension and repeat for reps.

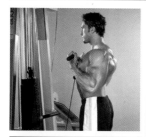

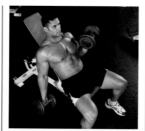

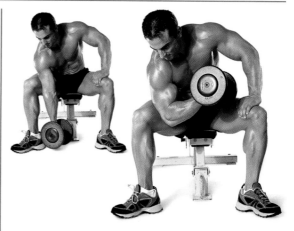

Standing Cable Curl

>> Take an underhand grip on a curl bar attached to a low pulley cable, arms extended. With abs tight, chest up and head straight, contract your biceps to curl the bar toward your chest, keeping your elbows at your sides. Hold and squeeze at the top, then slowly return the bar along the same path. Repeat for reps.

Incline Dumbbell Curl

>> Adjust an incline bench to 45–60 degrees. Sit back, feet flat on the floor, arms hanging at your sides, palms up. With shoulders back and upper arms in a fixed position perpendicular to the floor, curl the weights toward your shoulders. Squeeze your biceps hard at the top before slowly returning to the start.

Concentration Curl

>> Sit at the end of a flat bench. Bend over and grasp a dumbbell with an underhand grip, locking your working arm against your same–side inner thigh. Place your nonworking arm on the same side leg for balance. Moving only at your elbow, curl the weight as high as you can. Squeeze your biceps at the top before lowering the dumbbell back to the start.

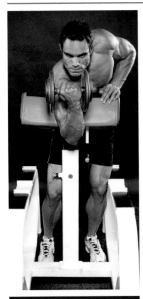

Dumbbell Scott Curl

» Grab a dumbbell and lean your chest against the angled side of a preacher bench, keeping your back tight and legs slightly bent. Make certain your armpit fits securely against the top of the pad, with your triceps pressed into the flat side of the bench. Place your nonworking hand on the bench for balance. Hold the dumbbell straight down towards the floor, with a palms-up (supinated) grip, your thumb wrapped around the handle. Keep your head in a neutral position, eyes focused forward. Curl the dumbbell up in a smooth arc, making sure to avoid using body English to get through the rep. Squeeze your biceps hard for a two-count before slowly lowering the dumbbells back to the starting position.

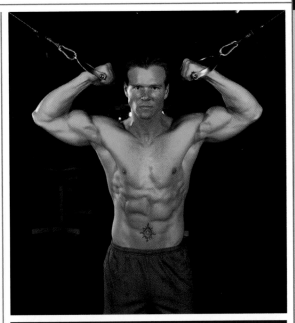

High-Cable Curl

» Stand in the middle of a cable crossover holding two D-handles attached to the high pulley cables. Keeping your elbows high, curl the D-handles toward the back of your head, behind your ears. Squeeze your biceps, then slowly return the handles to the start. Keep a slight bend in your arms at the start of each rep.

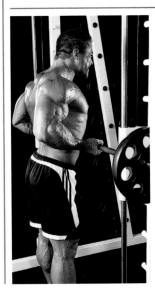

Smith Drag Curl

» Stand inside a Smith machine holding the bar in front of your upper thighs, with your chest up, shoulders back and eyes focused forward. Begin the move by pulling your elbows back as you curl the bar toward your upper abs/lower chest. As the name suggests, actually drag the bar up your torso as high as possible, keeping your elbows behind you. Slowly return the bar along the same path and repeat.

Machine Preacher Curl

» Place your upper arms against the pad snugly and grasp the handles. Curl as high as you can without your elbows leaving the pad, then lower to a point just before the weight stack touches down.

Cable Concentration Curl

» Sit at the end of a flat bench placed in front of a low pulley cable. Bend over and take an underhand grip on a D-handle, locking your working arm against your same-side inner thigh. Let the cable travel under your leg. Place your nonworking arm on the same side leg for balance. Moving only at your elbow, curl the handle as high as you can. Squeeze your biceps at the top before lowering the cable back to the start.

Dumbbell Preacher Curl

» Grab a dumbbell and lean your chest against the angled side of a preacher bench, armpit against the top of the pad. Grasp the bench with your nonworking hand for balance. Hold the dumbbell down toward the floor, palms-up grip, your thumb wrapped around the handle. Curl the dumbbell up in a smooth arc. Squeeze your biceps for a two-count before slowly lowering the weight back to the start.

TRICEPS

The beauty of the giant-set workout for triceps lies not just in its intensity but in its diversity. The lying triceps dumbbell extension that starts off the routine is a good overall triceps developer that works well for adding mass. The seated overhead dumbbell extension places more emphasis on the long head, followed by the dumbbell kickback, which is more of a shaping exercise that requires the use of lighter weights. The close-grip push-up hits the triceps' lateral heads especially well while utilizing higher reps (since you use only your bodyweight) for three high-intensity burnout sets. When doing giant sets, choose a first exercise that allows you to go heavy, then progress to lighter and lighter moves.

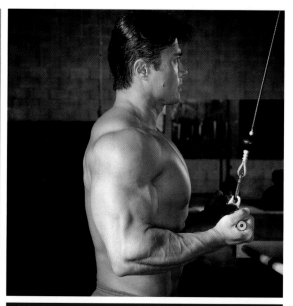

Reverse Grip Pressdown

» Stand in front of a high cable pulley and grasp the straight-bar attachment with an underhand grip. With your legs slightly bent, lean forward slightly at the waist and position your elbows close to your sides, as your bring your lower arms parallel to the floor. Flex your triceps and press the bar down toward the floor until your arms are fully extended. Squeeze your tris and hold for a brief count before returning to the start position.

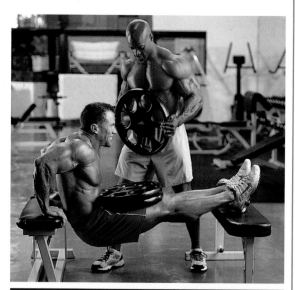

Weighted Bench Dip

» Put two benches a few feet apart and parallel to each other. Sit on the middle edge of one bench facing the other. Place your hands just outside your hips on the bench, cupping the bench with your fingers. Place your heels on the opposite bench, pressing yourself upward so that your body forms an "L" in the top position. After a partner places weight across your lap, slowly lower your glutes toward the floor until your arms form 90-degree angles. Pause, then force-fully press yourself back up to the start position.

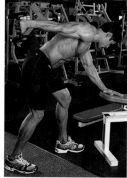

Dumbbell Kickback

» Grasp the rubber ball on the lower pulley cable, and align the working side shoulder with the pulley. Bend over until your torso is almost parallel to the floor. Raise your upper arm to parallel to your torso and keep it pressed into your side. Holding your upper arm in place, kick your lower arm straight back to full extension. Don't allow your elbow to drop as you return your lower arm to the start position.

#61 MASS-BUILDING

EXERCISE	SETS	REPS
Lying Triceps Extension	4	6, 8, 10, 12
Weighted Bench Dip	4	6, 8, 10, 12
Close-Grip Bench Press	4	6, 8, 10, 12
Pressdown	3	8, 10, 12

#62 BEGINNER'S

EXERCISE	SETS	REPS
Pressdown	4	10, 10, 12, 12
Dumbbell Kickback	3	10, 10, 10
Seated Overhead Cable Extension	3	10, 10, 10

#63 AT-HOME

EXERCISE	SETS	REPS
Close-Grip Push-Up	4	8, 10, 12, 20
Lying Triceps Dumbbell Extension	4	10, 12, 12, 20
Dumbbell Kickback	4	12, 12, 15, 20

#64 15-MINUTE WORKOUT

EXERCISE	SETS[1]	REPS
Standing Overhead Cable Extension	3	6, 10, 15
Reverse-Grip Pressdown	3	6, 10, 15
EZ-Bar Pressdown	3	6, 10, 15

#65 TRICEPS LONG HEAD PRIORITY

EXERCISE	SETS	REPS
45-Degree Lying Triceps Extension	4	10, 10, 12, 12
Seated Overhead Dumbbell Extension	4	8, 8, 10, 10
Weighted Bench Dip	4	10, 12, 15, 15
Pressdown	3	10, 10, 12

#66 TRICEPS LATERAL HEAD PRIORITY

EXERCISE	SETS	REPS
Close-Grip Bench Press	5	6, 8, 10, 10, 12
Rope Pressdown	3	8, 10, 12
Seated Overhead Dumbbell Extension	3	8, 10, 12

#67 GIANT-SET WORKOUT[2]

EXERCISE	SETS	REPS
Lying Triceps Dumbbell Extension	4	10, 10, 10, 10
Seated Overhead Dumbbell Extension	4	10, 10, 10, 10
Dumbbell Kickback	4	10, 10, 10, 10
Close-Grip Push-Up	4	to failure

#68 STRENGTH

EXERCISE	SETS[3]	REPS
Smith Close-Grip Bench Press	4	4, 4, 6, 8
Seated Overhead Cable Extension	4	4, 4, 6, 8
Straight-Bar Pressdown	4	4, 4, 6, 8

#69 GET RIPPED

EXERCISE	SETS[1]	REPS
Reverse-Grip Pressdown	5	10, 12, 12, 15, 20
Weighted Bench Dip	4	12, 12, 15, 15
Triceps Dip	4	to failure

#70 GET SUPER PUMPED

EXERCISE	SETS[1]	REPS
Lying Triceps Extension	4	10, 10, 30, 30
Seated Overhead Rope Extension	4	10, 10, 30, 30
Rope Pressdown	4	10, 10, 30, 30

[1] Rest no more than 30 seconds between each set.
[2] A giant set consists of four or more exercises performed consecutively without rest as a means to increase intensity and promote muscle growth. Do one set of each exercise back-to-back — that's one giant set. Rest three minutes between each giant set.
[3] Rest 2–3 minutes between each set.
Notes: The above workouts don't include warm-up sets. Unless otherwise noted, rest 60–90 seconds between all sets.

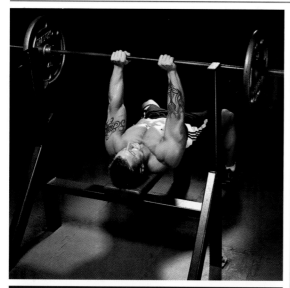

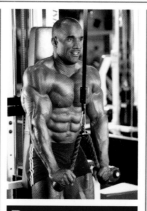

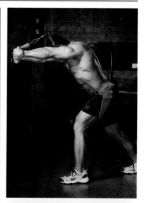

Close-Grip Bench Press

» Lie back on a flat bench with your feet on the floor. Grasp the barbell with a narrow (inside shoulder-width), overhand grip. Press the bar up slightly to unrack it and hold the bar above your chest with your arms extended. Lower the bar to your lower chest, keeping your elbows close to your body. Do not bounce the bar off your chest, but rather when the bar approaches an inch or so away from your chest, pause and press the bar back up to the starting position. Squeeze your triceps and chest at the top and repeat.

Rope Pressdown

» Stand in front of a high cable pulley and grasp the rope attachment with a neutral grip. Legs slightly bent, lean forward slightly at the waist and position your elbows close to your sides as you bring your lower arms parallel to the floor. Flex your triceps and press the bar down toward the floor until your arms are fully extended, pronating your hands at the bottom. Squeeze your tri's and hold for a brief count before returning to the start position.

Overhead Cable Extension

» Sit or stand in facing away from a low cable pulley. Grasp a straight bar or rope attachment with your arms at 90 degrees. Squeeze your triceps to press upward to full extension. Squeeze, the lower to the start.

45-Degree Lying Triceps Extension

» Lie face-up on a flat bench with your feet flat on the floor. Have a partner hand you a straight bar (or EZ-bar) and grasp it with an overhand grip. With your arms extended, hold the bar at a 45-degree angle above your head, back toward your spotter. Squeeze your triceps as you slowly lower the bar down toward the top of your head. When you reach a 90-degree angle in your elbows, pause for a moment, then forcefully extend your arms and press the bar back to the starting position.

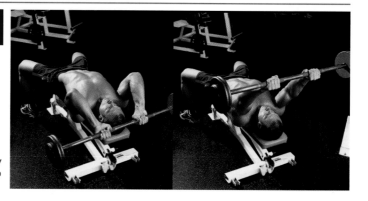

Seated Overhead Dumbbell Extension

» Sit erect on a low-back bench, feet flat on the floor. Grasp the inner plate of a dumbbell as your hold it overhead at full arm extension. Wrap your thumbs around the bar. Keep your head straight and lower back pressed into the pad. Bending only at your elbows and holding them in place alongside your ears, lower the weight behind your head until your arms form 90-degree angles. Hold for brief count, then press back up to full-arm extension and squeeze your triceps hard at the top.

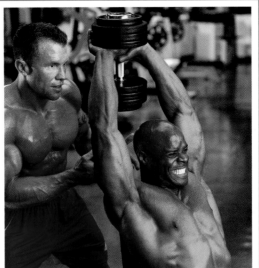

Seated Overhead Cable Extension

» Attach a rope to a high-cable pulley, then grasp it with a neutral, shoulder-width grip and face away from the stack. Take a step out with one foot and lean forward at the waist 30–45 degrees, keeping your abs tight, eyes forward, back straight and upper arms almost parallel to the floor. Moving only your lower arms, extend them out in front of you until your arms are parallel to the floor. Squeeze your triceps hard before returning to the start position

Smith Close-Grip Bench Press

» Lie back on a flat bench placed inside a Smith machine with your feet flat on the floor. Grasp the barbell with a narrow (inside shoulder–width), overhand grip. Rotate and press the bar up slightly to unrack it and hold the bar above your chest with your arms extended. Lower the bar to your lower chest, keeping your elbows close to your body. Do not bounce the bar off your chest, but rather when the bar approaches an inch or so away from your chest, pause and press the bar back up to the starting position. Squeeze your triceps and chest at the top and repeat.

Close-Grip Push-Up

» Lie face-down on the floor in a push-up position, placing your hands a few inches apart. Raise your body by extending your arms and coming up on your toes. With your forehead facing the floor and your abs pulled in, lower your body by bending your elbows. Stop the motion when your chest taps the floor and reverse to the start.

Triceps Dip

» Grasp the dip bars with your arms extended. Keep your upper body upright as much as possible. Keep your elbows tight to your sides as you bend them to lower your body down toward the floor. Press your hands into the bars to extend your arms and raise your body back up to the start.

FOREARMS

With one of their main duties being to assist in gripping, the forearms are some of the most functional muscles we have. If you lack grip strength, you'll never reach your full potential in the weight room, especially on exercises such as deadlifts and rows. Unfamiliar with the exercises in the grip-strength workout? For the horizontal cable hold, stand in the middle of a cable crossover station with D-handles set to shoulder level, select a heavy weight, grasp the handles and stand in an iron cross position for the allotted time; for the plate pinch, hold two 10-pound plates in each hand down at your sides and pinch the plates together with your fingers (progress to heavier plates as you grow stronger); and for the straight-arm hang, simply hang from a pull-up bar with your arms straight, hands shoulder-width apart, for as long as you can.

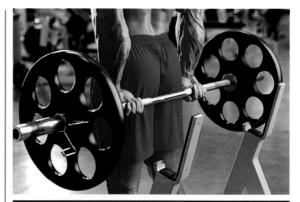

Behind-the-Back Wrist Curl

» Stand holding a barbell behind your back with an overhand, pronated grip. Allow your thumbs to be on the same side as your fingers. Let the barbell roll to the end of your fingers and thumbs, then curl the barbell upward as high as possible. Squeeze your forearms, then return to the starting position.

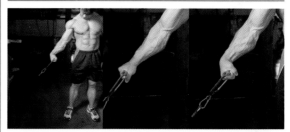

Standing Cable Wrist Curl

» Stand next to a low cable pulley, holding a D-handle in one hand, arm extended. Using just your wrist, curl the cable upward squeezing your forearms, then return to the starting position.

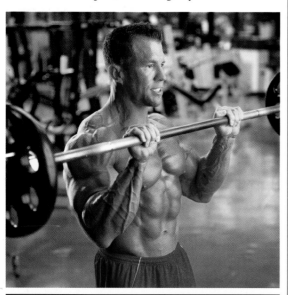

Reverse Curl

» Stand holding a barbell with an overhand grip, arms extended. Keep your abs tight, chest up and head straight. Contract your biceps and forearms to curl the bar toward your chest, keeping your elbows at your sides. Hold and squeeze your biceps and forearms at the top, then slowly return the bar along the same path.

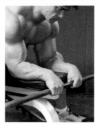

Reverse Wrist Curl

» Sit at the end of the bench, holding a barbell with a narrow, overhand grip. Allow your lower arms to rest on the bench, with only your hands off the edge. Curl the bar upward, squeezing your forearms, then return to the starting position.

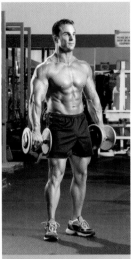

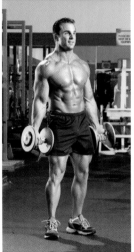

Zottman Curl

» Stand holding a pair of dumbbells with a palms-down, pronated grip. Curl the dumbbells up toward your shoulders. Squeeze, then rotate the dumbbells so your palms face upward. Slowly lower the weights to your sides. Repeat the sequence for reps.

Barbell/ Dumbbell Wrist Curl

» Sit at the end of a bench with your fore-arms flat on the bench, while you hold a barbell in your hands. Allow the barbell to roll to your fingers, then use your wrists to curl the bar-bell back to the start.

Horizontal Cable Hold

» Stand in the middle of a cable crossover and hold D-handles at shoulder level with both hands. Your arms should form a "T". Continue to hold against resistance until failure.

Plate Pinch

» Place a plate between your fingers and thumb and hold for as long as possible. Increase weight as you progress in strength.

Straight-Arm Hang

» Find an overhead bar and hop up and grasp the bar with a shoulder-width grip. Steadily hang for as long as possible. After a brief rest, repeat.

Reverse Scott Curl

» Hold a barbell with an overhand, pronated grip on the flat side of a preacher bench. Using just your forearms, curl the barbell upward as high as possible, then slowly lower to the start.

#71 MASS-BUILDING

EXERCISE	SETS	REPS
Reverse Curl	4	6, 8, 10, 12
Hammer Curl	4	8, 10, 10, 12
Barbell Wrist Curl	4	6, 8, 10, 12
Behind-the-Back Wrist Curl	3	8, 10, 12

#72 BEGINNER'S

EXERCISE	SETS	REPS
Dumbbell Wrist Curl	3	10, 10, 10
Standing Cable Wrist Curl	3	10, 10, 10

#73 AT-HOME

EXERCISE	SETS	REPS
Dumbbell Reverse Curl	4	8, 10, 12, 20
Zottman Curl	3	10, 12, 20
Hammer Curl	3	12, 12, 15
Dumbbell Wrist Curl	2	10, 10

#74 GRIP STRENGTH

EXERCISE	SETS	REPS
Horizontal Cable Hold	4	30 seconds
Plate Pinch	3	30 seconds
Straight-Arm Hang	3	to failure

#75 GET SUPER PUMPED

EXERCISE	SETS*	REPS
Reverse Scott Curl	4	10, 10, 30, 30
Reverse Curl	4	10, 10, 30, 30
Reverse Wrist Curl	4	10, 10, 30, 30

* Rest no more than 30 seconds between each set.
Notes: The above workouts don't include warm-up sets. Unless otherwise noted, rest 60–90 seconds between all sets.

CALVES

In most beginner's workouts, the exercises aren't too different from those in an advanced lifter's routine; instead, volume and intensity tend to be somewhat lower for the beginner. Basic mass- and strength-building moves are good for trainees of all levels, and you'll continue to use seated and standing calf raises indefinitely in your lower-leg training. For beginners, the key is to take this time to master technique so you don't form bad habits, especially with a bodypart as stubborn as the calves. When training calves, no matter the exercise, be sure to go all the way up onto your toes at the top of each rep and go all the way down at the bottom for a stretch. Using a full range of motion is a must for turning your calves into cows.

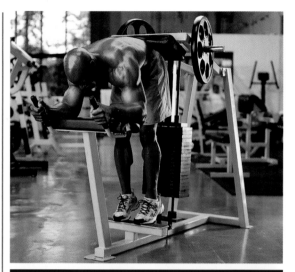

Donkey Calf Raise

» Step into a donkey calf machine with the balls of your feet on the foot platform and your upper glutes/lower back secured under the pad. Allow your forearms to rest on the arm pad and grasp the handles. Press up onto your toes, and squeeze before lowering your heels toward the floor as low as possible. Repeat.

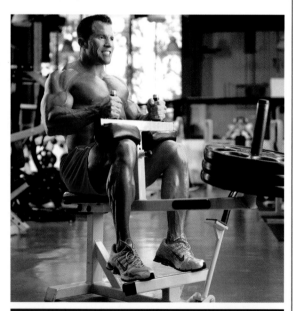

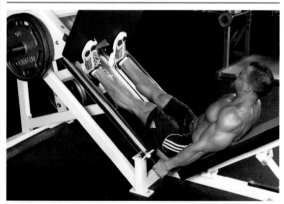

Seated Calf Raise

» Sit at a seated calf machine, with the balls of your feet on the foot rests and the pads secured across your lower quads. Press up with your calves to unrack it, then lower your heels to the floor. After a good stretch, press up onto your toes as high as possible, squeeze and repeat.

Leg Press Calf Raise

» Sit in a leg press machine and place the balls of your feet at the bottom of the platform, heels off the edge. Do not unrack the safety bars. Press through the balls of your feet and squeeze your calves hard. Slowly lower your toes downward and repeat.

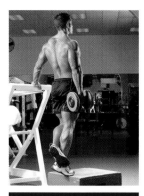

Dumbbell Calf Raise

>> Stand on a box or platform with one foot, grasping a dumbbell in one hand and holding a stable surface with the other hand. Allow your working heel to travel toward the floor, then press upward onto your toes as high as possible. Repeat.

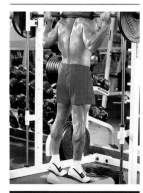

Smith Calf Raise

>> Stand inside the Smith with the balls of your feet on a short platform. With the bar across your upper back, let your heels travel toward the floor for a good stretch, then press up onto your toes as high as possible. Repeat.

Seated Dumbbell Calf Raise

>> Sit on the end of a bench, with the balls of your feet on a short platform as you hold dumbbells across your lower quads. Press up with your calves, then lower your heels to the floor. After a good stretch, press up onto your toes again as high as possible and squeeze. Repeat for reps.

Seated Smith Calf Raise

>> Sit on the end of a bench inside a Smith machine, with the balls of your feet on a short platform as you hold the bar across your lower quads. Press up with your calves, then lower your heels to the floor. After a good stretch, press up onto your toes as high as possible and squeeze.

Power Rack Calf Raise

>> Inside a power rack, set the safeties high (around shoulder level). Place the bar across your upper back. The balls of your feet can be on a short platform or simply flat on the floor. Press up onto the balls of your feet, then lower your heels toward the floor. The bar should touch the safeties at the bottom of each rep.

#76 MASS-BUILDING

EXERCISE	SETS	REPS
Standing Calf Raise	5	8, 10, 12, 15, 25
Seated Calf Raise	5	8, 10, 12, 15, 25
Leg Press Calf Raise	3	10, 15, 20

#77 BEGINNER'S

EXERCISE	SETS	REPS
Standing Calf Raise	2	15, 15
Seated Calf Raise	2	15, 15

#78 AT-HOME

EXERCISE	SETS	REPS
One-Leg Dumbbell Calf Raise	4	10, 10, 15, 15
Seated Dumbbell Calf Raise	4	10, 10, 15, 15

#79 GIANT-SET WORKOUT[1]

EXERCISE	SETS	REPS
Smith Calf Raise	4	15, 15, 20, 20
Seated Smith Calf Raise	4	15, 15, 20, 20
Donkey Calf Raise	4	15, 15, 20, 20
Leg Press Calf Raise	4	15, 15, 20, 20

#80 GET SUPER PUMPED

EXERCISE	SETS[2]	REPS
Donkey Calf Raise	4	10, 10, 30, 30
Leg Press Calf Raise	4	10, 10, 30, 30
Power Rack Calf Raise	4	10, 10, 30, 30

[1] A giant set consists of four or more exercises performed consecutively without rest as a means to increase intensity and promote muscle growth. Do one set of each exercise back-to-back — that's one giant set. Rest three minutes between each giant set.
[2] Rest no more than 30 seconds between each set.
Notes: The above workouts don't include warm-up sets. Unless otherwise noted, rest one minute between all sets.

ABS

For most people, the lower abs are by far the most difficult region of the midsection to carve out, since this area typically attracts more bodyfat as opposed to just under your pecs. A clean diet is crucial to great lower abs, but the muscles also need to be fully developed to show through.

All three exercises in the lower abs priority workout entail crunching the pelvis up and toward the rib cage, the opposite motion of the standard crunch, in which the pelvis remains stationary and the shoulders and chest move, targeting the upper abs. Our prescribed rep ranges (10–20) aren't astronomical; it doesn't take sets of 50–100 to get abs, as long as you perform each exercise slowly and under control, squeezing the full benefit out of every muscle contraction.

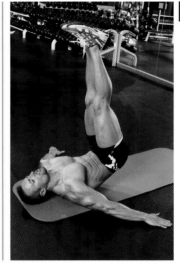

Hip Thrust

» Lie face-up on the floor with your hands extended at your sides. Lift your feet up so your legs are roughly perpendicular to the floor. Contract your abs to raise your hips and glutes straight up off the ground to push your feet toward the ceiling. Hold this position for a count before lowering your glutes back to the floor.

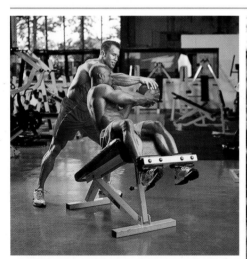

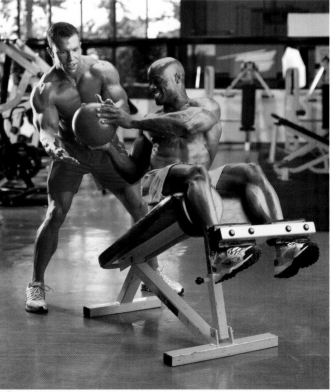

Decline Medicine-Ball Twist

» Sit on the decline bench in a half sit-up position (your lower back shouldn't touch the bench) and hold the medicine with both hands straight above you. With your arms locked in that position, rotate your torso to the right until your right arm is about parallel to the floor as you hand the ball to your partner. Rotate then retrieve the ball from your partner on the other side. Work in both directions.

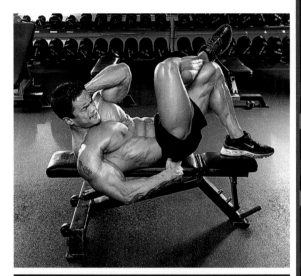

Crossover Crunch

» Lie on the floor or on a flat bench with one knee crossed over the opposite leg. Crunch your body up and across, taking your elbow to the opposite knee. Squeeze and return to the start, then repeat on the other side. Once to each side equals one rep.

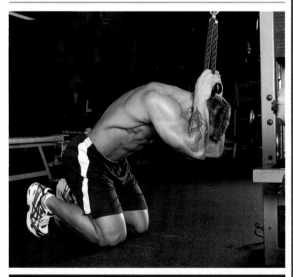

Kneeling Cable Crunch

» Kneel in front of a cable machine and grasp a rope attachment with both hands. With your lower arms aside your head, crunch down, taking your elbows to the floor. Pause, then slowly return to the start.

#81 BEGINNER'S

EXERCISE	SETS	REPS
Crunch	2	15, 15
Reverse Crunch	2	15, 15

#82 AT-HOME

EXERCISE	SETS	REPS
Double Crunch	2	20, 20
Crossover Crunch	2	15, 15
Scissor Kick	2	10, 10

#83 10-MINUTE WORKOUT

EXERCISE	SETS*	REPS
Hanging Leg Raise	2	15, 15
Kneeling Cable Crunch	2	15, 15
Decline Medicine-Ball Twist	2	10, 10

#84 UPPER ABS/OBLIQUES PRIORITY

EXERCISE	SETS	REPS
Decline Medicine-Ball Twist	2	15, 15
Lying Cable Crossover Crunch	2	15, 15
Machine Crunch	2	15, 15

#85 LOWER ABS PRIORITY

EXERCISE	SETS	REPS
Hanging Knee Raise	2	15, 15
Hip Thrust	2	10, 10
Scissor Kick	2	20, 20

* Perform these three exercises back-to-back without resting between sets (called a tri-set). Rest one minute between each tri-set.
Notes: The above workouts don't include warm-up sets. Unless otherwise noted, rest 30–60 seconds between all sets.

NOTE: For much more on ab training, including a five-week program, see chapters 4 and 5.

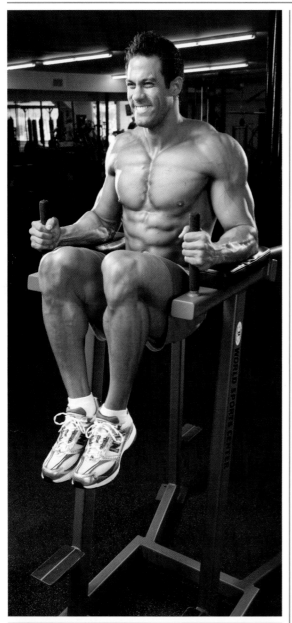

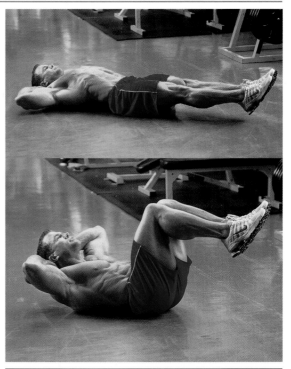

Double Crunch

>> Lie on the floor with your hands cupped gently behind your head and your legs almost completely straight and raised a few inches off the floor. Simultaneously bring your knees to your torso while crunching your upper body toward your legs. Squeeze in the middle, then return to the start and repeat. Don't let your feet touch the floor between reps.

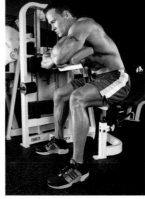

Machine Crunch

>> Sit inside an ab machine with your arms across the pad. With your feet flat on the floor, flex your abs to crunch forward, moving the pad towards your knees. Squeeze and hold, then return to the start. Don't allow the weight plates to touch down between reps.

Hanging Knee Raise

>> Either hanging from an overhead bar or supported on a vertical bench (as shown), contract your abs to bring your knees as high as possible in front of you. Pause and squeeze momentarily, then slowly lower your legs to the start position and repeat.

Hanging Leg Raise

» Grasp an overhead bar and hang freely. Keeping your legs straight, raise them straight up in front of you as high as possible without using momentum. Pause as long as possible, then return to the start position and repeat.

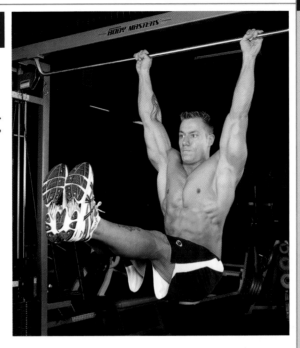

Scissor Kick

» Lie on your back with your arms by your sides, palms facing down, legs extended with a slight bend in your knees. Lift your heels off the floor about 6 inches, then make small, rapid, alternating up-and-down scissorlike motions as you lift each leg about 45 degrees into the air and lower each until your heel is a few inches off the floor.

Lying Cable Crossover Crunch

» Lie face-up on the floor, knees bent about 60 degrees and feet flat. Cross your left ankle over your right knee. Hold a rope attachment, ends at each side of your head. Curl up as high as you can, bringing your shoulder blades off the floor, simultaneously trying to bring your right elbow across your body toward your left knee. Repeat for reps, then switch positions and complete reps to the opposite side.

Reverse Crunch

» Lie on the floor or reversed on a decline bench, grasping the ankle pads with your hands. Contract your abs to bring your knees toward your chest, allowing your glutes to gently lift off the bench. Squeeze, return your legs to the start and repeat for reps.

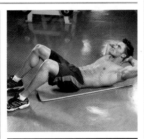

Crunch

» Lie face-up on the floor with your legs bent and your feet flat. Place your hands behind your head with your fingertips touching to support your head and your elbows out to your sides. Slowly curl your upper body upward, raising your shoulder blades off the floor as your raise your chest and shoulders toward the ceiling, squeezing your abs before returning to the start.

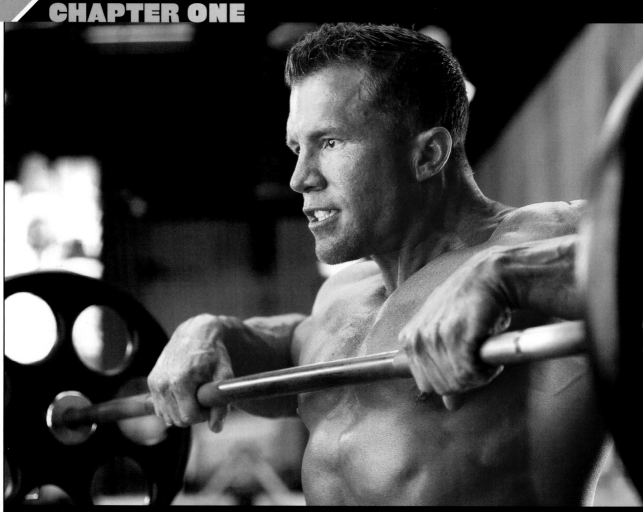

THE WEIDER PRINCIPLES

Build the perfect routine — or make any workout better — with these 24 tried-and-true training principles, collected by the Master Blaster himself, Joe Weider

In the preceding 85 workouts, we've provided many ways to improve every major bodypart. Each one relies on the strength of the chosen exercises, set selection and rep ranges to target every muscle group.

However, as with any training program, you can take what we've given and tweak it, depending on your level of experience and need for higher intensities to blast through any training plateau. The Weider Principles, a list of weightlifting truisms gathered and honed by the father of bodybuilding, Joe Weider, have stood the test of time. These 24 principles, which we've divided into three categories, have guided us for decades in our program design. We highly recommend that you use them, too, as you learn and advance your muscle-building efforts.

PROGRAM DESIGN

CYCLE TRAINING Devote portions of your training year to specific goals for strength, mass or getting cut. This can help decrease your risk of injury and add variety to your routine. Cycle periods of high intensity and low intensity to allow for recovery and spur new gains.

ECLECTIC TRAINING Incorporate a diverse selection of variables, such as set, rep and exercise schemes, into your workout. Utilize both mass-building multi-joint movements and single-joint exercises.

INSTINCTIVE TRAINING Experiment to develop an instinct as to what works best for you. Use your training results along with past experiences to constantly fine-tune your program. Go by feel in the gym: If your biceps just don't *feel* like they've recovered from the last workout, do another bodypart that day instead.

MUSCLE CONFUSION Constantly change variables in your workout — number of sets, number of reps, exercise choice, order of exercises, length of your rest periods — to avoid getting in a rut and slowing growth.

INTENSITY BOOSTERS

CONTINUOUS TENSION Don't allow a given muscle to rest at the top or bottom of a movement. Control both the positive and negative portions of a rep and avoid momentum to maintain constant tension throughout the entire range of motion.

FLUSHING TRAINING Train one bodypart with multiple exercises (3–4) before you train another. The "flushing" is your body sending a maximum amount of blood and muscle-building nutrients to that area to best stimulate growth.

HOLISTIC TRAINING Use numerous training techniques (low and high reps, faster and slower speeds, and alternate exercises) to stimulate maximum muscle fibers. Don't always approach exercises with the same 6- to 10-repetition sets; try lightening the load and going for 20 reps in some training sessions to build endurance-related muscle fibers.

ISOLATION TRAINING This is a technique designed to work individual muscles without involving adjacent muscles or muscle groups. A pressdown for triceps (rather than a close-grip bench press) is an example of an isolation movement.

ISO-TENSION Between sets (or even between workouts), flex and hold various muscles for 6–10 seconds, keeping them fully contracted before releasing. Competitive bodybuilders use this technique to enhance their posing ability through increased muscle control.

(Principles continued on page 58)

BODY**SLAM**

GET FIT FAST WITH THIS 40-MINUTE FULL-BODY WORKOUT

Sure, you'd like to go to the gym 4–6 days a week for an hour or so a pop, but real life doesn't always work out as we plan.

When you find yourself short on time, or if you're in an extremely busy stretch and can't make it to the gym more than twice a week, you may want to hit your whole body in one fell swoop. This regimen gives you the tools to do just that.

The key to this workout is that it contains one exercise for each bodypart that hits the greatest amount of muscle fibers, so you get the most bang for your buck. Notice how each movement is a basic, core exercise for the respective muscle group, as opposed to a strict isolation move. To speed things along, you'll rest only 30 seconds between each set and do only 1–2 sets per exercise. Even though you'll get in and out of the gym in about 40 minutes, it's crucial that you make the most of every set, taking each one to failure at close to the suggested number of reps to promote hypertrophy. To avoid injury, do 1–2 light warm-up sets before your working sets for each exercise.

Ideally, when training for muscle size or strength, you should perform bodypart routines on different days and train with higher volume. That said, employ this routine only when you have a time crunch, as it won't maximize the gains you'd see when training longer and more frequently. But when "one of those weeks" is upon you, this 40-minute full-body gauntlet should keep your training goals on track.

#86 THE BODY**SLAM** WORKOUT

BODYPART	EXERCISE	SETS	REPS
CHEST	Incline Barbell Press	2	8, 12
BACK	Bent-Over Row	2	8, 12
LEGS	Barbell Squat	2	8, 12
SHOULDERS	Overhead Dumbbell Press	2	8, 12
TRAPS	Barbell Shrug	1	12
BICEPS	Close-Grip Barbell Curl	1	12
TRICEPS	Lying Triceps Extension	1	12
CALVES	Donkey Calf Raise	1	25
ABS	Double Crunch	1	to failure

Notes: The above workout doesn't include warm-up sets. Rest 30 seconds between all sets.

Chatting on your cell while spotting: the ultimate gym faux pas.

SINS OF THE GYM

CHANCES ARE THAT IF YOU'RE NOT GROWING, YOU'RE MAKING ONE OF THESE SIX CRITICAL TRAINING MISTAKES

Take a look around the gym and you can easily spot the beginners: guys doing barbell curls in rhythm with a pelvic thrust, and a lot of bouncing out of the hole in squats and bench presses. Too bad they're not the only ones making mistakes. In fact, intermediate- and advanced-level bodybuilders also commonly make critical errors in their workouts, ultimately slowing their progress. And there are also some universal bad habits that we gym rats commit from time to time that could be a burden to those around us.

1) UNBRIDLED ENTHUSIASM

You want to get big, but Rome wasn't built in a day, and you won't be, either. Doing hours of biceps curls won't make your arms grow any faster — and could be counterproductive. "Enthusiasm is good if you've never worked out before and you're starting a new program, but doing too much too fast won't do your body any good," sas Adam Garett, a certified personal trainer at Bally Total Fitness in Oakland Park, Florida.

"Beginners often try to do every exercise for every bodypart, but that enthusiasm needs to be tempered because hormones that break down muscle quickly start rising. Expect to hit your body hard for 45–60 minutes total, about 30 minutes for a given muscle group; you can't maintain the intensity very long when your energy levels are trailing off. Also, remember that training stimulates the process of muscle breakdown, but growth occurs after your workout during your recovery period, which is aided by good nutrition." This also applies to overambitious lifters who get carried away with volume and intensity.

2) NOT LEARNING EVERY VARIATION OF A GIVEN MOVE

Although you may know how to perform every exercise in your workout with textbook technique, you will build thicker, denser muscles if you learn how to do each of its variations. For instance, if you're doing standing dumbbell lateral raises for your middle delts, also try doing the move from a seated position or one arm at a time while standing. Other alternatives include using cables for raises, both in front and behind your back, and doing the movement with one arm as you lean to the side by gripping a vertical post with your opposite hand.

Virtually every exercise can be tweaked. "Knowing how to do a particular move a number of ways can be helpful when there's a line in front of ou for a given piece of equipment, but each and every variation also works the muscle a little differently, and this helps build the muscle more fully," Garett explains.

3) NOT MAKING THE MOST OF YOUR TIME AT THE GYM

If you're a gym member, then you're paying for the resources to build a better body. So why waste time when you're there? Too often, you'll see lifters — regardless of their level of experience — spending a great deal of their time resting in the gym.

Whether it's taking a longer-than-necessary breather between sets, leaving their racked and towel-shrouded equipment for a bathroom break or rubbernecking to get a look at the hottie on cardio row, extended rest can be detrimental to your progress. Go to the gym to work — use your couch at home to lounge and recover.

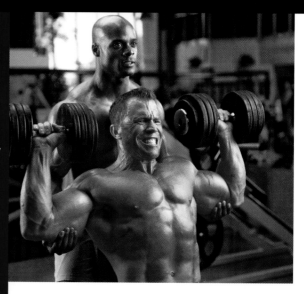

4) NOT PUTTING YOUR MIND TO WORK

Once you've been training for a while, your muscles adapt and you no longer make strength and size gains the way you did as a beginner. While switching up exercises can help, it's time to rethink your approach and try some extraordinary methods to jump-start serious muscle growth.

"Listen to your body and focus on the pump and feeling the muscle work, worrying less about sets and reps," Garett says. "Consciously make the decision to challenge yourself by doing exercises you hate, or by using other high-intensity methods such as rest-pause or cycled training that you haven't tried before."

5) NOT PRACTICING THE "LITTLE THINGS"

If there's one thing advanced lifters know, it's sore joints and aches and pains. These problems don't just go away when you're lifting heavy day after day. The more progress you make, the more important it is to pay attention to all the things you skipped as a beginner, Garett says. This includes making sure you do a thorough warm-up, performing rotator-cuff stretches and exercises, stretching afterward (especially your lower back and hamstrings to help prevent low-back pain) and knowing the difference between good and bad pain. Over the long term, such little things will prove huge.

6) NOT PAYING ATTENTION

If you're lucky enough to have a training partner, make sure you use that to your advantage, not as a hindrance to your progress. Studies show that those who lift in the presence of others have a tendency to push around more weight than they would lifting alone. And after your partner helps you push through your heavy sets, be sure to return the favor. Marginalizing your duties as a reciprocating spotter by going through the motions, chatting or looking away will keep your partner from reaching his goals and is an open invitation for injuries. Besides, you'll have time to socialize postworkout.

MUSCLE PRIORITY Hit your weakest bodypart first in a workout or bodypart split, when you can train with more weight and intensity because your energy level is higher.

PEAK CONTRACTION Squeeze your contracted muscle isometrically at the endpoint of a rep to intensify effort. Hold the weight in the fully contracted position for up to two seconds at the top of an exercise.

PROGRESSIVE OVERLOAD To continue making gains, your muscles need to work harder in a progressive manner from one workout to the next. During most of your training cycle, try to increase your weights each session, do more reps or sets, or decrease your rest periods between sets.

PYRAMID TRAINING Incorporate a range of lighter to heavier weights for each exercise. Start light with higher reps (12–15) to warm up the muscle, then gradually increase the weight in each successive set while lowering your reps (6–8). You could also reverse the procedure — moving from high weight and low reps to low weight and high reps, aka a reverse pyramid.

ADVANCED TRAINING TECHNIQUES

SUPERSETS Perform sets of two exercises for the same or different muscle groups back-to-back with no rest in between.

TRI-SETS Perform three consecutive exercises for one muscle group in nonstop sequence.

GIANT SETS Four or more exercises for one muscle

group performed in back-to-back fashion without rest in between.

BURNS Continue a set past the point at which you can lift a weight through a full or even partial range of motion with a series of rapid partial reps. Do this as long as your muscles can move the weight, even if only a few inches.

CHEATING Use momentum (a slight swing of the weight) to overcome a sticking point as you fatigue near the end of a set. While doing heavy barbell curls, for example, you might be able to perform only eight strict reps to failure. A subtle swing of the weight or a slightly faster rep speed may help you get 1–2 additional reps. For advanced bodybuilders only.

DESCENDING OR DROP SETS After completing your reps in a heavy set, quickly strip an equal amount of weight from each side of the bar or select lighter dumbbells. Continue to do reps until you fail, then strip more weight off to complete even more reps.

FORCED REPS Have a training partner assist you with reps at the end of a set to help you train past the point of momentary muscular failure. Your training partner will lift the bar with just enough force to get you past the sticking point.

NEGATIVES Resist the downward motion of a very heavy weight. For example, on the bench press, use a weight that's 15%–25% heavier than you can typically handle, and fight the negative as you slowly lower the bar to your chest. Have your partner assist with the positive portion of the rep.

PARTIAL REPS Do reps involving only a partial range — at the top, in the middle or at the bottom — of a movement.

PRE-EXHAUSTION You pre-exhaust a muscle with a single-joint exercise before performing a multijoint movement. In leg training, you can start with leg extensions (which target the quads) before a set of squats (which also work the glutes and hamstrings).

REST-PAUSE Take brief rest periods during a set of a given exercise to squeeze more reps out of a set. Use a weight you can lift for 2–3 reps, rest as long as 20 seconds, then try for another 2–3 reps. Take another brief rest and go again for as many reps as you can handle, and repeat one more time.

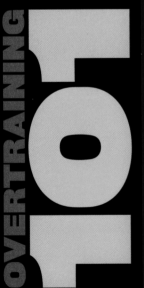

OVERTRAINING 101

HERE'S HOW TO IDENTIFY WHETHER YOUR BODY IS OVERTRAINED AND HOW TO BUST OUT OF YOUR RUT ONCE YOU'RE THERE

WHAT TO WATCH FOR

Fatigue	Drop in blood pressure
Increased resting heart rate	Irritability
Digestion problems	Depression
Decrease in strength	Joint pain
Decrease in muscle mass	Sleeping troubles

WHAT TO DO WHEN OVERTRAINED

1) Reduce training volume, intensity and/or frequency, or take an extended break of 1–2 weeks
2) Loosen normal dietary restrictions
3) Engage in activities outside the gym
4) Start supplementing with protein (20 grams of whey immediately preworkout and 40 grams of whey or a whey-casein mix immediately postworkout) and glutamine (5 grams with breakfast, pre- and postworkout, and before bed)
5) Return to the gym with a restructured routine that incorporates fewer intensity techniques, more moderate loads and more rest between sessions

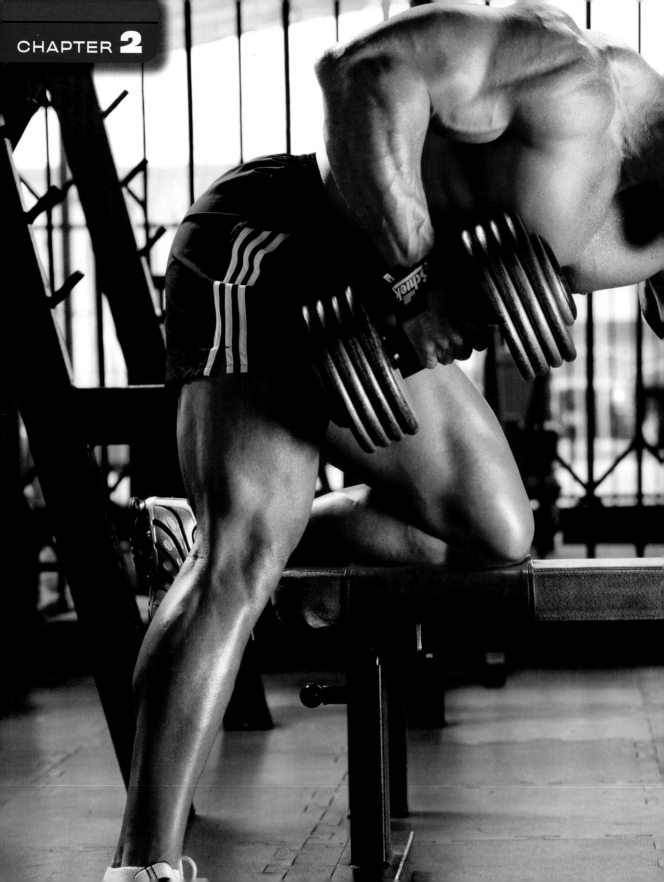

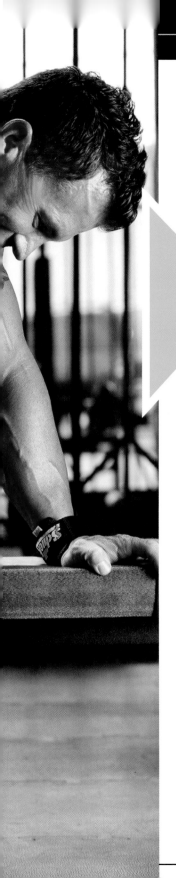

Fast-Forward Your Fat Loss Part 1

Ready for a nine-week program that will help you burn off that unwanted flab and get fitter, leaner and stronger than ever before? These next two chapters deliver just that, starting with a supercharged five-week workout and cardio plan detailed in the following six pages, and an intense four-week training regimen presented in Chapter 3 to bring it all together.

Whether you've picked up this book in the winter, spring summer or fall, it's never a bad time to start yourself on the road to the body you've always wanted — no question, any time of year is a good time for a lean physique. And if you have a special event like a vacation, reunion or wedding coming up, this will provide the perfect way to get ready. So what are you waiting for? Get to the gym, tighten up your trouble spots, and build muscle mass and definition simultaneously.

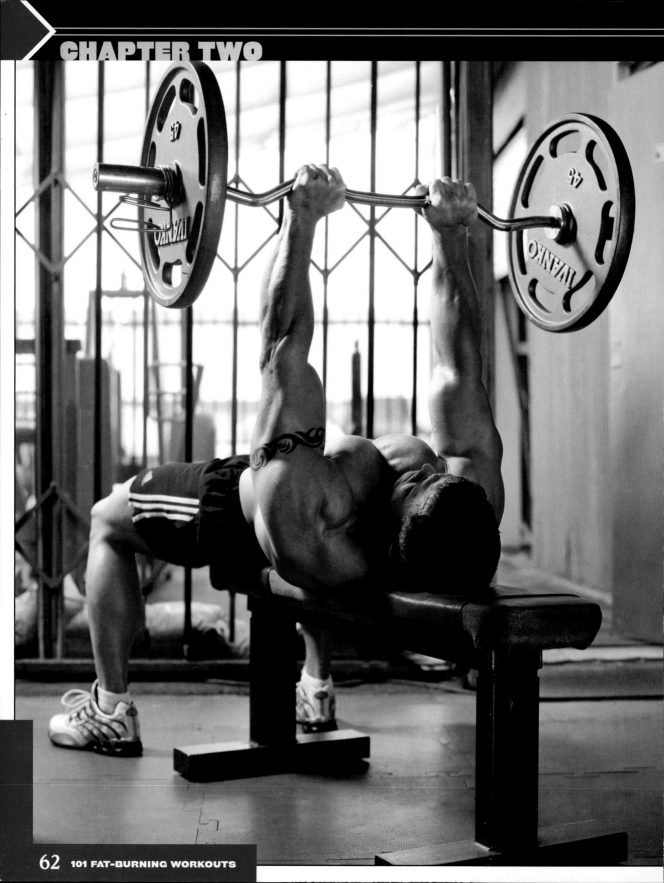

YOUR LEAN MACHINE

If you're currently slugging through your typical workouts, you'll immediately notice one change when you undertake this program. Your training intensity will increase, not necessarily in terms of using heavier weights but rather in applying advanced techniques that take your muscles past the point of failure. This strategy isn't for the faint of heart; it's for those who are ready to dig in and work to achieve their goals. Stick with it and, combined with appropriate cardio and diet components, the end result will be well worth your sweat and your time.

The goals of the program are to reduce bodyfat and develop muscle definition. You'll weight-train four days a week in the first three weeks, and increase that frequency to five days a week for the final two weeks leading up to the final month (outlined in Chapter 3).

The degree of change you'll see will be a result of the intensity you apply; in other words, if you slack off, you'll limit your ultimate potential. Consistency is your key to success. Given the shortened timetable, it's imperative that you don't skip workouts.

Sets and reps are based on a light-to-heavy pyramid system; in most cases, your first set is a warm-up with a light weight. Successive sets use heavier resistance, so be sure to choose a weight that allows you to reach muscle failure at the rep indicated.

The given rep ranges will allow you to craft new muscle *only* if you choose weights that challenge you. Remember, building muscle during a get-ripped program is important — muscle is metabolically active and burns calories, even at rest, so the more muscle you add, the more efficient your body will become at burning excess calories. The advanced training techniques and shortened rest periods will help you build that fantastic physique you're looking for.

WEEKS 1–3

In the first three weeks, you'll split your bodyparts into three workouts. Remember to follow all the rules of

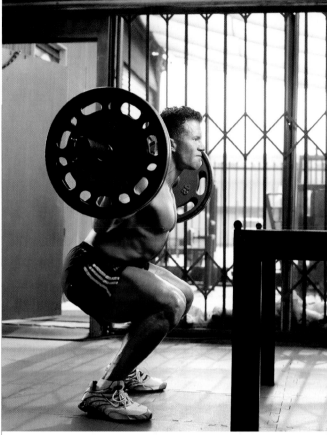

good lifting: Use correct form and controlled speed, squeeze at the point of peak contraction, lower under control and avoid momentum. Also be aware of the length of your rest periods between sets; stick with 60 seconds, no more. If your rest periods become too long, you start training more like a powerlifter and less like a bodybuilder, in essence working against the stated purpose of this get-lean routine.

In addition, we've selectively chosen advanced training techniques to use with the heaviest sets of certain exercises for each bodypart — for example, you might do drop sets for back and forced reps for chest. Some techniques require an attentive spotter; if you don't have one, substitute another technique.

WEEKS 4–5

Here, we pump up the intensity and workload by splitting muscle groups into two workouts instead of three. Move from set to set and exercise to exercise more quickly, and rest only 45 seconds between sets. Finally,

FAST-FORWARD WORKOUTS

WEEKS 1-3

#87 Workout 1: Chest + Back + Abs

EXERCISE	SETS	REPS	ADVANCED TECHNIQUE
Bench Press	4	15,12,8^1,8^1	Forced Reps
Incline Dumbbell Press	3	12,8,8	
Pec-Deck Flye	2	12,12	
Bent-Over Row	4	12,10,8,8	
Seated Cable Row	2	8^1,8^1	Drop Sets
Back Extension	2	20,20	
Pull-Up	3	to failure	
Hanging Leg Raise	2	15,15	
Crunch	2	20,20	
Decline Twisting Crunch	2	15,15	

#88 Workout 2: Legs + Calves + Abs

EXERCISE	SETS	REPS	ADVANCED TECHNIQUE
Squat	4	15,12,10,8	
Hack Squat	3	12,10,10	
Leg Extension	3	15,12^1,10^1	Drop Sets
Romanian Deadlift	3	12,10,10	
Lying Leg Curl	2	12,10^1	Partial Reps
Standing Calf Raise	3	15,15,15	
Decline Weighted Crunch	2	10,10	
Straight-Leg Crunch	2	15,15	
Hanging Oblique Knee Raise	2	12^2	

#89 Workout 3: Shoulders + Traps + Arms + Abs

EXERCISE	SETS	REPS	ADVANCED TECHNIQUE
Overhead Dumbbell Press	3	15,10,8	
Dumbbell Lateral Raise	2	10^1,10^1	Drop Sets
Bent-Over Lateral Raise	2	10,10^1	Drop Sets
Barbell Shrug	3	12,10,8	
Close-Grip Bench Press — superset with^1 —	3	12,10,8	Supersets
Rope Pressdown	3	10,10,10	Supersets
Barbell Curl — superset with —	3	12,10,10	Supersets
Dumbbell Hammer Curl	3	10,10,10	Supersets
Reverse Crunch	2	15,15	
Machine Crunch	2	15,15	

WEEKS 4-5

#90 Workout 1: Legs + Back + Calves

EXERCISE	SETS	REPS	ADVANCED TECHNIQUE
Leg Extension^1	3	12,10,10	Pre-Exhaust
Smith Machine Squat	3	12,10 ,10	Drop Sets
Leg Press	3	10,10,8	
Glute-Ham Raise	3	12,10,10	
Seated Leg Curl	3	12,8^1,8^1	Drop Sets
Dumbbell Row	3	12,10,8	
Seated Cable Row	2	10^1,10^1	Drop Sets
Back Extension	2	20,20	
Pull-Up	3	to failure	
Standing Calf Raise	3	15,15,15	
Seated Calf Raise	2	15,15^1	Partial Reps

#91 Workout 2: Chest + Shoulders + Arms + Abs

EXERCISE	SETS	REPS	ADVANCED TECHNIQUE
Incline Barbell Press	3	15,10^1,8^1	Forced Reps
Flat-Bench Dumbbell Press	3	10,10,10	
Pec-Deck Flye	2	15,15^1	Partial Reps
Machine Overhead Press	3	15,10^1,8^1	Drop Sets
Cable Lateral Raise	2	10^1,10^1	Drop Sets
Reverse Pec-Deck Flye	2	10,10	
Weighted Bench Dip	3	10,10^1,8^1	Drop Sets
Lying Triceps Extension	2	10,10	
Barbell Curl	3	12,10,8	
EZ-Bar Preacher Curl	2	12,10^1	Forced Reps
Hanging Knee Raise^3	3	15,15,15	
Cable Crunch	3	15,15,15	

^{1} Apply advanced technique listed.
^{2} Lifting knees to each side once equals one rep.
^{3} Hold medicine ball between knees.

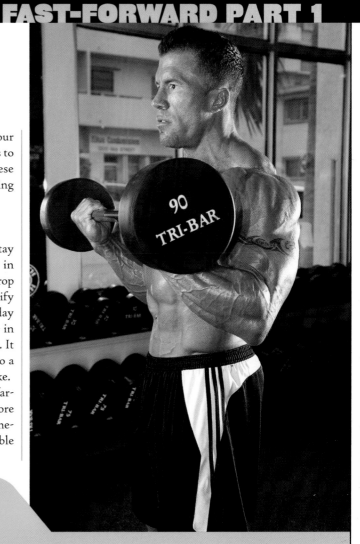

use advanced techniques more frequently to take your training past failure. The goal in these two weeks is to kick up your metabolism, so bring a towel — if these workouts don't make you sweat, you're not expending enough effort.

THE LONG VIEW

This program isn't easy, nor is it supposed to be. To stay on track, keep your goal consistently and clearly in mind. Is it to lose 3 inches off your midsection? Drop your bodyfat percentage into the single digits? Identify your goal, take measurements of where you are today and post that information in a conspicuous place — in the office, on the fridge, wherever you'll see it often. It also helps to hang a picture of yourself today next to a picture from a magazine of what you want to look like.

Dream big, but be realistic: You can have a far-improved physique in a couple months, but more dramatic changes take time. Remember, this nine-week program is just a start — but what an incredible start it will be.

PROGRAM GUIDELINES

>> **Always begin** with a 5- to 10-minute warm-up on the cardio equipment of your choice.

>> **During weeks 1–3,** train Monday, Tuesday, Thursday and Friday (with Wednesday off), so you'll complete the three workouts in four days and start the cycle again on the fifth. Take 60 seconds to rest between sets.

>> **During weeks 4–5** train five days a week, performing the two workouts on consecutive days, then taking a day off; repeat until the two weeks are up. Cut your rest periods by 15 seconds but still strive to lift the same amount of weight for the same number of reps.

>> **After your first warm-up set** for most bodyparts, choose a weight that allows you to reach the target rep range at muscle failure. Your last few reps should be difficult.

>> **Extend your set** where indicated with advanced training principles. These include:

Supersets — Do exercises back-to-back with no rest.

Forced reps — A training partner provides assistance after you reach failure, allowing you to complete a couple of extra reps.

Drop sets — Once you reach muscle failure, quickly reduce the weight by 20%–30% and continue repping until you reach failure again. At that point, do one more drop set to failure to ratchet up your intensity even further. Select your weights ahead of time for convenience.

Partial reps — Once you reach muscle failure, complete several additional reps by powering through a very short range of motion.

Pre-exhaust — Perform a single-joint exercise before the compound movement to prefatigue the targeted muscle group.

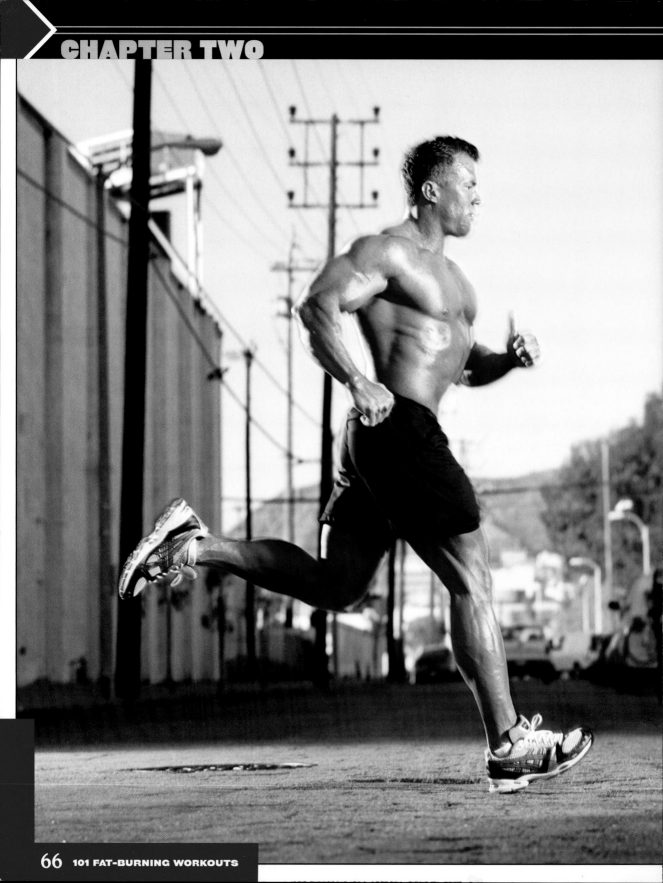

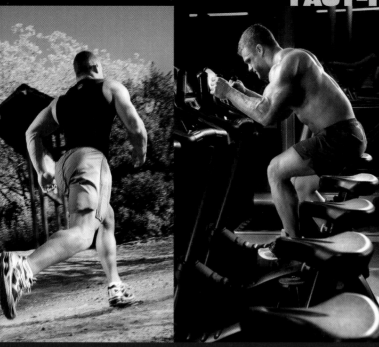
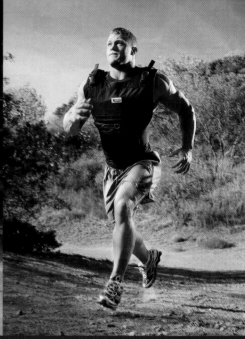

THE FAST-FORWARD CARDIO PROGRAM

>> **To burn the optimal amount of bodyfat, you need cardio.** (Sorry, cardio haters.) But no one said it had to be boring. Choose any of the following five cardio options, doing it either when you go to the gym for your weight workout (just be sure to do cardio after weights) or at another time of day, such as first thing in the morning on an empty stomach. In weeks 1–3, do cardio 4–5 times a week; in weeks 4–5, do cardio 5–6 times a week.

1 INTERVAL TRAINING A

Equipment: Treadmill, elliptical, recumbent bike or rower. **Workout:** Five-minute warm-up; 25 minutes at a 1:1 high:low intensity ratio (for instance, one minute sprinting on a treadmill, followed by one minute at a jogging pace); five-minute cool-down.

2 INTERVAL TRAINING B

Equipment: Treadmill, elliptical or outdoor track **Workout:** Five-minute warm-up; 25 minutes at a 1:2 high:low intensity ratio; five-minute cool-down.

3 SPRINTS

Location: Indoor or outdoor track. **Workout:** Jog two laps as a warm-up; perform 4x400-meter sprints with two-minute walking recovery between each; jog two laps as a cool-down.

4 LONG, STEADY-PACE CARDIO

Equipment: Treadmill, elliptical or recumbent bike. **Workout:** Go at a challenging pace for 45–60 minutes; the pace should be difficult enough that you break a sweat, but you should still be able to pass the "talk test" (you are able to speak without becoming breathless).

5 HILL REPEATS

Location: Either on a treadmill with an incline feature or an outdoor hill (choose a steeper incline if you have a higher fitness level). **Workout:** Ten-minute jogging warm-up; perform 10 50-yard sprints up an incline with one-minute walking recovery between each sprint (or a brisk walk/jog back down the hill); 10-minute flat-terrain jogging cool-down.

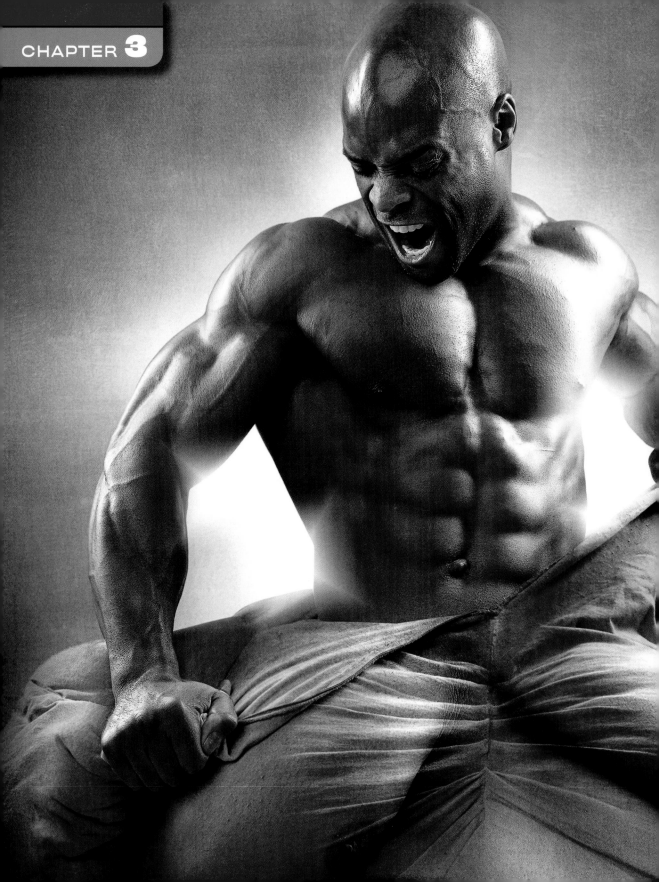

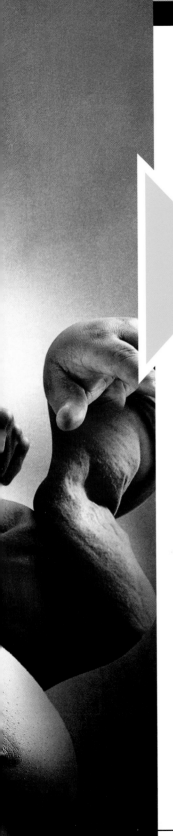

Fast-Forward Your Fat Loss Part 2

Now that you're five weeks in, how do you feel? You should be energized, and ready to do exactly what the guy is doing at left — stripping away your old physique with this four-week sprint to the finish of your nine-week journey.

The following program is truly a synthesis of benefits, bringing together high-volume lifting and ultra-intense cardio: It's a mix of high- and low-rep training plus interval-based cardio and longer, steady-state exercise. That's because one without the other might have you burning some bodyfat, but not nearly as much as you're capable of when they are employed in combination.

Over the next four weeks, the workouts will be tough and the month might seem long, but at the end of the program you'll surely realize why you did it. You'll have burned lots of blubber and your abs will be showing. Not a bad combination at all.

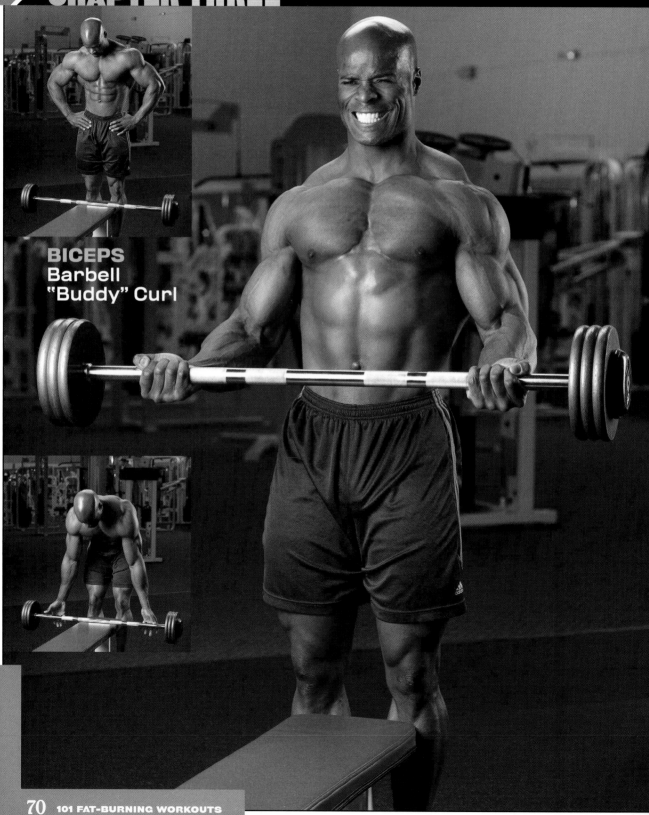

BICEPS
Barbell
"Buddy" Curl

In this program, you'll train six days a week (Monday through Saturday), each workout consisting of both lifting weights and cardio. You'll do more or less the same routines every week, and with the high volume and intense nature of the workouts, this plan will be very effective since your body will still be adapting to the stress placed on it through the fourth week. The specific exercises, sets, reps and exercise durations to use can be found later in the chapter, but here's a general rundown of what each day will entail.

DAY 1 | MONDAY

The training week will start with a high-volume arm workout and a heavy-duty cardio session, performed in that order. The weightlifting will consist of three exercises each for biceps and triceps.

For biceps, start with what's called a buddy curl. First, select a weight with which you'll reach failure at around 10 reps. Do one rep, then pass the bar to your training partner. He'll do his rep, then hand the bar back to you for two reps. Hand it back to him for two reps, then it's back to you for three reps, and so on. Do this in one-rep increments until you reach 10 reps on your last set. (If you don't have a lifting partner, set the bar down on a bench between sets and rest as long as it would take someone else to do the same number of reps.) This method is great for adding volume and intensity to your workout, which are hallmarks of this program. Perform all the other exercises for biceps and triceps in straight-set fashion.

As you'll notice, nearly every exercise (one exception being buddy curls) will consist of 3–4 sets of reps ranging from 6–20. Go heavy on your first set to hit the low end of this range, then progressively lighten the load so you're doing 20 reps by your third or fourth set. This makes your muscles work with heavy, moderate and light weights, all in the span of minutes for each exercise, which keeps your body guessing and less likely to adapt to a constant resistance. Moreover, the heavy sets help you maintain muscle in the midst of the clean dieting and extensive cardio you'll undertake, both of which can strip away muscle along with the fat if you're not careful.

The cardio routine planned for Mondays will be repeated on Thursdays and Fridays each week, and it represents the most intense sessions you'll do over the course of the program. It consists of three elements: 1) one-minute intervals of jumping rope, 2) 30-second intervals using a heavy rope and 3) 25 reps of bench jumps (50 total jumps over and back). Perform this circuit 10 times through for an intense cardio workout that'll melt away bodyfat. Each week, increase the volume of each move: Add a minute to each jump rope interval, 30 seconds to each heavy rope bout and 10 reps to each set of bench jumps.

DAY 2 | TUESDAY

Your second session of the week is leg day. And we'll be honest: It's high-volume, very intense work. The workout consists of basic compound exercises such as squats and leg presses, and three different supersets to hit the largest muscles of the lower body — the quads, glutes and hamstrings. A couple of novel exercises — the barbell crawl and jump squat — are added to the mix to provide a further shock to the body.

INTENSIVE FAT-LOSS TRAINING SPLIT

DAY	BODYPART(S) TRAINED
1	Arms and cardio (intense)
2	Legs and cardio (easy)
3	Cardio (easy, long), abs and calves
4	Chest, shoulders and cardio (intense)
5	Back, traps and cardio (intense)
6	Cardio (easy, long), abs and calves
7	Rest

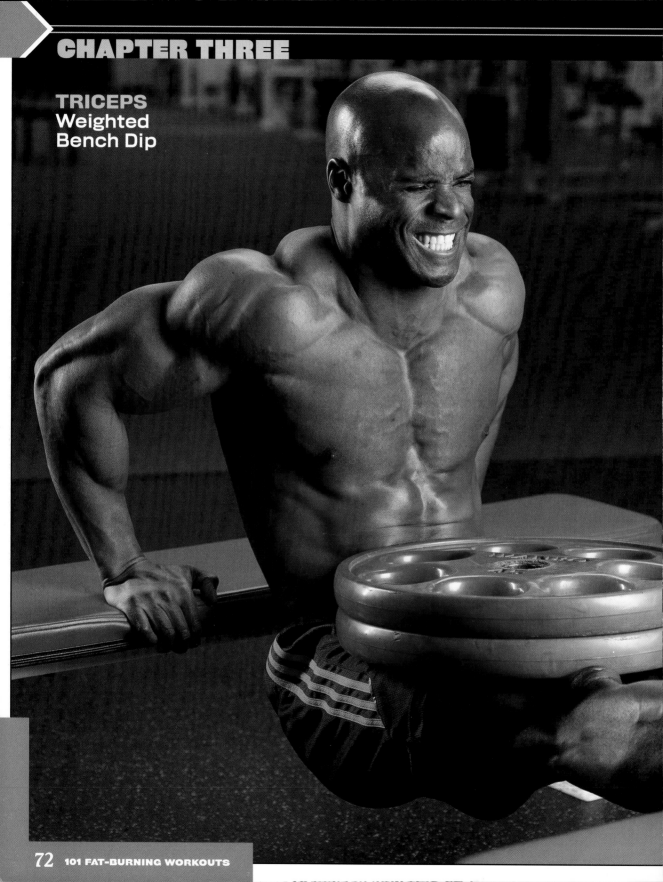

TRICEPS
Weighted
Bench Dip

Because your legs will no doubt be exhausted after performing 10 total movements for the lower body, you'll do a relatively easy cardio session immediately afterward. Again, you'll jump rope, but this time alternate jumping for one minute at an easy pace with resting one minute for 40 minutes (i.e., 20 minutes of actual jumping).

DAYS 3 + 6 | WEDNESDAY + SATURDAY

In each of these two training days, you will perform cardio first, followed by a short ab and calves workout. The cardio session (either a walk on a treadmill or stair-stepper) will be low in intensity and long — *two hours* long, to be exact. This serves as a drastic change of pace from the high-intensity cardio work you do on Monday, Thursday and Friday, and that's just the point. Your body will burn more fat by training at both high and low intensities.

The lifting on these days will be minimal, only abs and calves, with six sets total for each. Feel free to keep your rest periods short between sets (30–45 seconds) to move the workout along quickly.

DAY 4 | THURSDAY

Chest and shoulders are on tap for Thursdays, followed by the same cardio workout on Mondays. The exercises for pecs and delts are mostly basic, compound movements to hit the most muscle fibers possible to maximize calorie-burning. The volume is elevated (five exercises for chest, three for shoulders) to burn more calories during the workout and keep your metabolism elevated afterward.

DAY 5 | FRIDAY

Back and traps are the focus on Fridays, followed by the jump rope/bench jump cardio routine from the Monday and Thursday workouts. Train your back with high volume (four exercises) and fundamental exercises such as dumbbell deadlifts and T-bar rows.

For traps, in addition to dumbbell shrugs, you'll do the strongman exercise known as the farmer's walk (see page 77). This is considered a trap exercise because the upper traps will likely be the first muscles to succumb to exhaustion. (To ensure that your hands and forearms don't go first, use wrist straps.) But make no mistake, the farmer's walk involves myriad other muscles, from the upper back to the legs, making it a great calorie-burner that's ideal for this program.

And there you have it — the perfect combination of no-nonsense lifting and fat-blasting cardio. For the next four weeks, you'll subject your body to a multitude of training intensities and durations — the best of both worlds. Get ready to get lean in a hurry.

#92 DAY 1 | ARMS

EXERCISE	SETS	REPS
Biceps		
Barbell "Buddy" Curl	2	55[1]
Incline Cable Curl	3–4	6–20
Dumbbell Preacher Curl	3–4	6–20
Triceps		
Weighted Bench Dip	3–4	6–20
Triceps Pressdown	3–4	6–20
Standing Overhead Cable Extension	3–4	6–20

CARDIO

EXERCISE	DURATION/REPS
Jump Rope	1 minute
Heavy Rope	30 seconds
Bench Jump	25 reps[2]

>> Perform these exercises as a circuit 10 times.
>> During Weeks 2–4, increase your jump rope time by one minute each week, increase the heavy rope time by 30 seconds and increase your bench jumps by 10 reps. By Week 4, you should be doing four minutes of jumping rope, two minutes of heavy rope and 55 reps of bench jumps per circuit.

[2] Jumping over the bench and back is one rep.

[1] Select a weight that causes you to fail at around 10 reps. Do one rep, then rest one second or as long as it takes your partner to do one rep. Then do two reps, resting as long as it takes your partner to do two reps, and so on until you've reached 10 reps. That's one set.

CARDIO
Bench
Jump

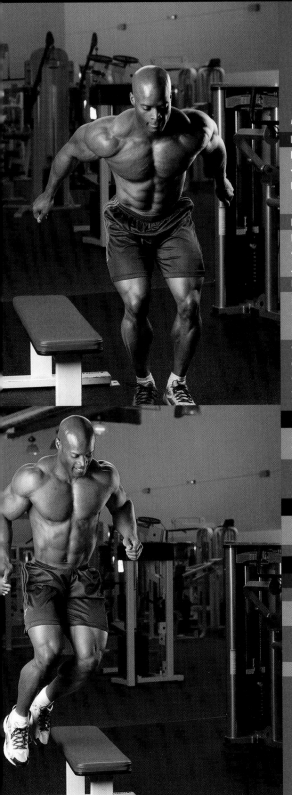

#93 DAY 2 | LEGS

EXERCISE	SETS	REPS
Barbell Squat	3–4	6–20
— superset with —		
Barbell Crawl*	3–4	40–60-foot walk after each set
Leg Press	3–4	6–20
Leg Extension	3–4	6–20
— superset with —		
Jump Squat	3–4	6–20
Romanian Deadlift	3–4	6–20
Lying Leg Curl	3–4	6–20
— superset with —		
Bodyweight Jump Squat	3–4	20

* Immediately after each set of squats, place a short, empty bar across your back, squat down and walk approximately 20–30 feet. Then stop, turn around and return to your starting point.

CARDIO

JUMP ROPE 1 minute on, 1 minute off for 40 minutes (amounts to 20 minutes of jumping rope and 20 minutes of rest)

#94 DAY 3 | ABS + CALVES

CARDIO

TREADMILL OR STAIR-STEPPER Two hours at low intensity (50%–60% of max heart rate)

ABS + CALVES

EXERCISE	SETS	REPS
Abs		
Hanging Leg Raise	3	to failure
Machine Crunch	3	10–12
Calves		
Standing Calf Raise	3	20
Seated Calf Raise	3	20

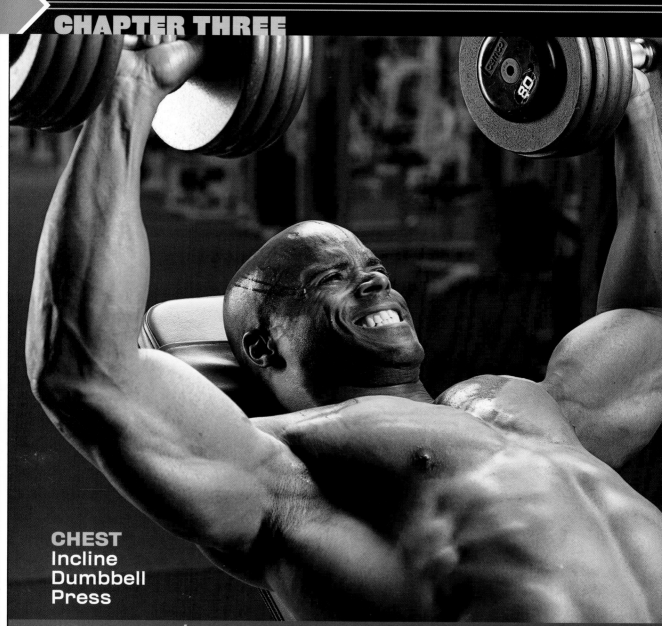

CHEST
Incline
Dumbbell
Press

#95 DAY 4 | CHEST + SHOULDERS

EXERCISE	SETS	REPS
Chest		
Incline Dumbbell Press	3–4	6–20
Incline Dumbbell Flye	3–4	6–20
Bench Press	3–4	6–20
Pec-Deck Flye	3–4	6–20
Smith Machine Decline Press	3–4	6–20
Shoulders		
Overhead Dumbbell Press	3–4	6–20
Cable Lateral Raise	3–4	6–20
Bent-Over Cable Lateral Raise	3–4	6–20

CARDIO

EXERCISE	DURATION/REPS
Jump Rope	1 minute
Heavy Rope	30 seconds
Bench Jump	25 reps*

>> Perform these exercises as a circuit 10 times.
>> During Weeks 2–4, increase your jump rope time by one minute each week, increase the heavy rope time by 30 seconds and increase your bench jumps by 10 reps. By Week 4, you should be doing four minutes of jumping rope, two minutes of heavy rope and 55 reps of bench jumps per circuit.

* Jumping over the bench and back is one rep.

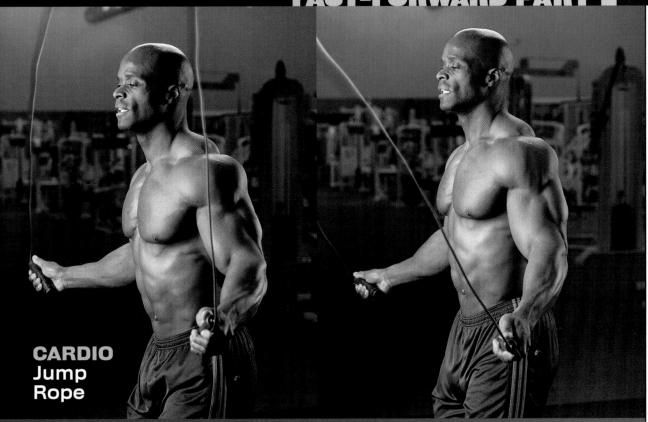

CARDIO
Jump
Rope

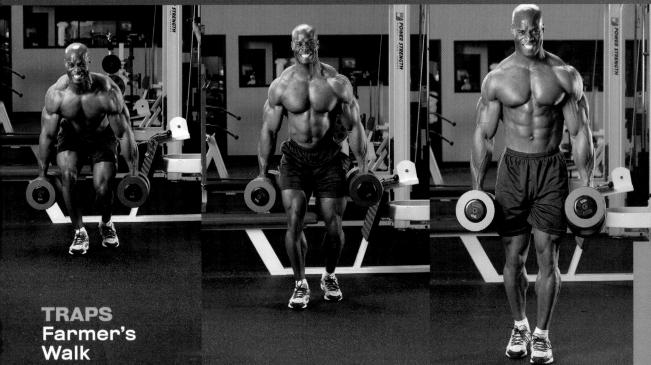

TRAPS
Farmer's
Walk

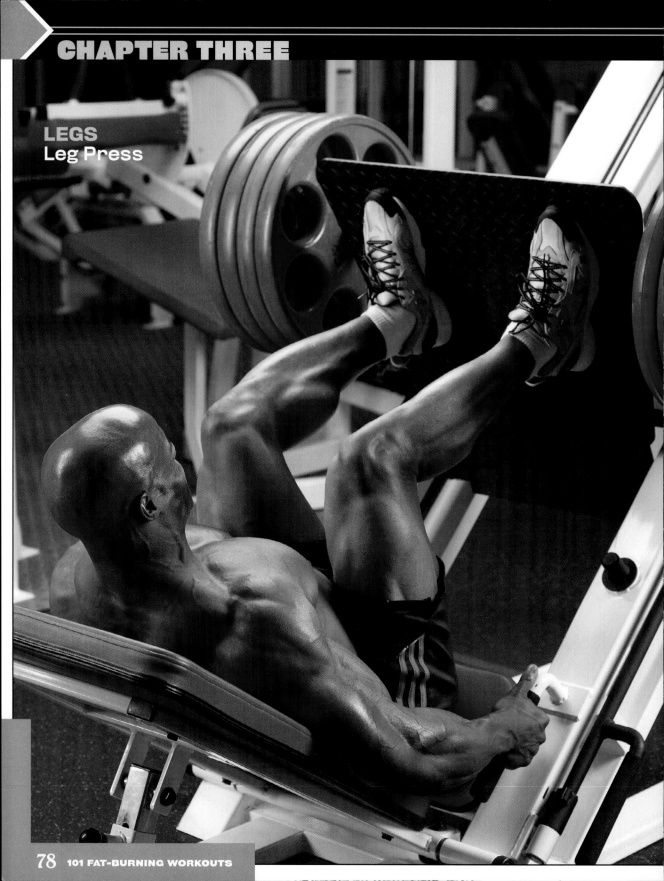

LEGS
Leg Press

LEGS
Barbell Crawl

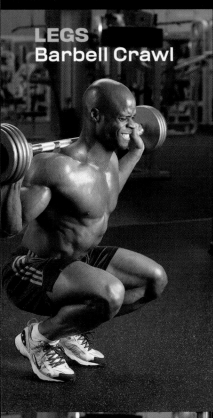

#96 DAY 5 | BACK + TRAPS

EXERCISE	SETS	REPS
Back		
Dumbbell Deadlift	3–4	6–20
T-Bar Row	3–4	6–20
Straight-Arm Lat Pulldown	3–4	6–20
Seated Row	3–4	6–20
Traps		
Farmer's Walk[1]	3–4	to failure
Dumbbell Shrug	3–4	6–20

[1] Select a weight that matches your 8- to 10-rep max on dumbbell shrugs (a relatively heavy weight). Hold the weights at your sides and walk approximately 20–30 feet. Stop, turn around and return to the start. Continue until you can no longer hold on to the weights due to upper trap fatigue.

CARDIO

EXERCISE	DURATION/REPS
Jump Rope	1 minute
Heavy Rope	30 seconds
Bench Jump	25 reps[2]

>> Perform these exercises as a circuit 10 times.
>> During Weeks 2–4, increase your jump rope time by one minute each week, increase the heavy rope time by 30 seconds and increase your bench jumps by 10 reps. By Week 4, you should be doing four minutes of jumping rope, two minutes of heavy rope and 55 reps of bench jumps per circuit.

[2] Jumping over the bench and back is one rep.

#97 DAY 6 | ABS + CALVES

CARDIO

TREADMILL OR STAIR-STEPPER Two hours at low intensity (50%–60% of max heart rate)

ABS + CALVES

EXERCISE	SETS	REPS
Abs		
Double Crunch	3	to failure
Decline Medicine-Ball Twist	3	15
Calves		
Donkey Calf Raise	3	20
Seated Calf Raise	3	20

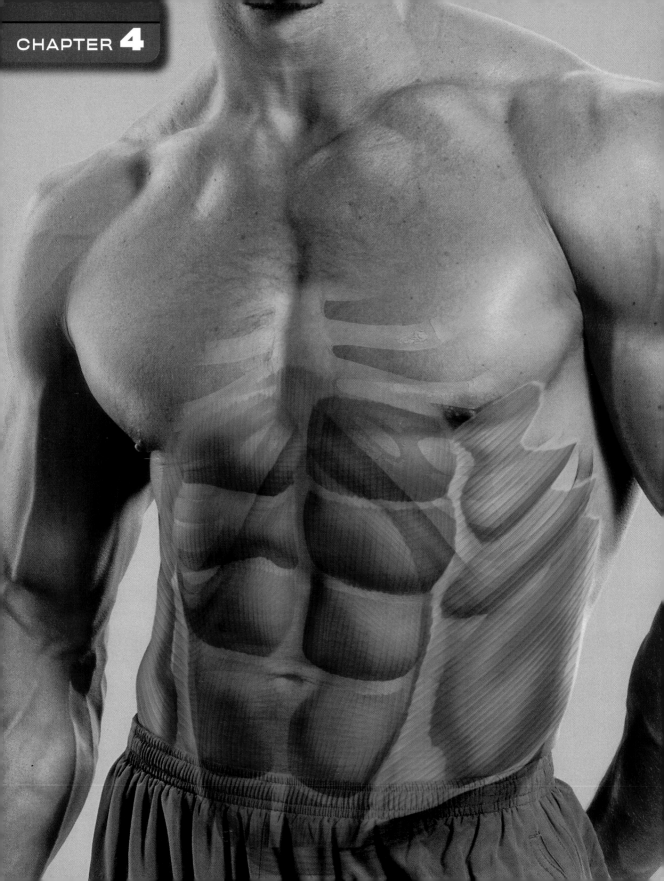

Ab Training 101

Pretend for just a moment that your midsection is a terrain you're trying to navigate. You'd like to explore a number of different regions, but you're not quite sure of the best way to go about it. After all, when it comes to the abdominals in particular, there are all sorts of conflicting opinions about how to traverse it most effectively and find the path to the ultimate six-pack.

Random wandering just won't do if you want to find the most reliable route between A and B (B being strong, well-defined abdominals). What you really need is the ab version of a high-tech GPS — something that will tell you how to arrive at your destination the quickest way possible.

That's where this chapter comes in. Think of the following six pages as your very own "Abdominal Positioning System," telling you what areas to train, when to train them and how — essentially eliminating the risk of getting lost or making any wrong turns along the way.

CHAPTER FOUR

ROUTE 6 (PACK)

The four muscles that make up what are generally called the abdominals are the:

1) rectus abdominis
2) internal obliques
3) external obliques
4) transverse abdominis

Without question, the best ab program is one that incorporates exercises for all these areas.

If you train abs more often than other bodyparts, you're not alone. Most people who give their abs the attention they deserve train them 3–5 times per week, although they may work other major bodyparts (chest, back, legs, etc.) 1–3 times per week. Reason being, the abs are postural muscles that stay flexed for long periods to support the spine. As such, they have a higher percentage of slow-twitch muscle fibers than other bodyparts and require more regular training for adequate stimulation.

The rep range you choose to work within is critical to the development of your abs and their appearance when your bodyfat is low. Using your own body-weight as resistance and keeping your reps between 15 and 30, for example, will help you maintain a flat, lean midsection, giving the impression of a smaller waist. If you want your abs to grow so you can see them better, you'll need to include weighted exercises using a cable station or a light weight plate or dumb-bell to help build them up. Selecting exercises is easy — choose a total of four moves every time you train abs, one for each of the different areas.

With ab training, timing is crucial: Always hit abs last in your workout. You don't want them to be fatigued before training other bodyparts, such as back or legs, because you want your abs and core to be strong and fresh to sustain the intra-abdominal pressure necessary to protect your spine.

So let's look at each region of the abs, dissecting their anatomy, location and function. We'll also review some of the best exercises you can do to get the kind of washboard midsection you want.

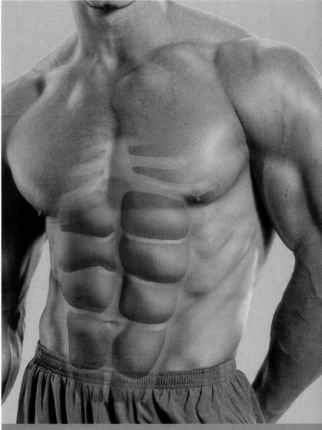

REGION 1
RECTUS ABDOMINIS

>> Even though the six-pack appears to be several individual muscles, the rectus abdominis is really only one. Running vertically from your sternum to your pelvis, the rectus is a thin sheath of muscle. While we'll discuss exercises for your upper and lower abs, note that they're all part of one muscle. That said, you can still emphasize the upper and lower portions of the rectus with specific movements.

The rectus abdominis facilitates the standard crunching motion — moving your rib cage toward your pelvis. It can also be trained in the opposite direction — bringing your pelvis to your rib cage — which we refer to as a reverse crunching motion.

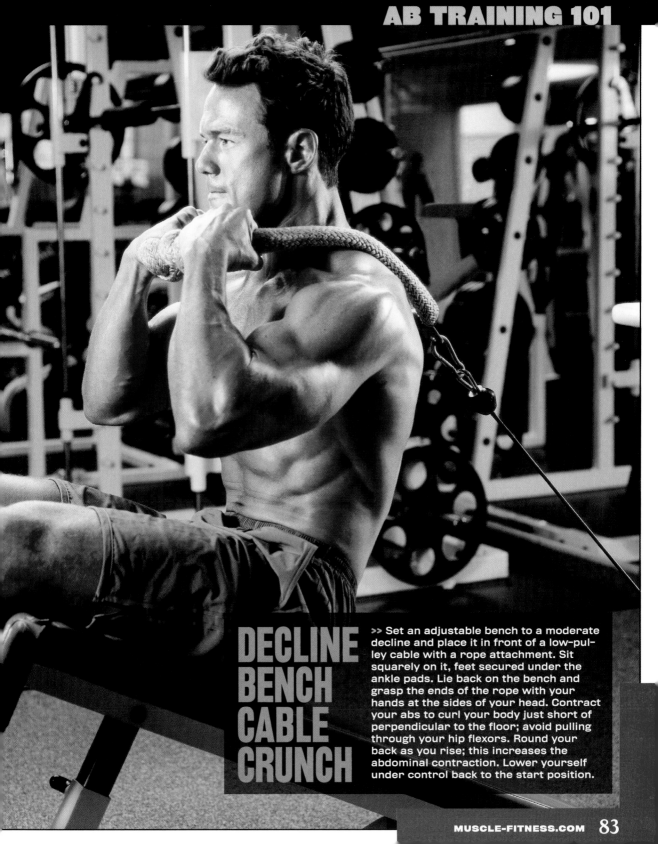

DECLINE BENCH CABLE CRUNCH

>> Set an adjustable bench to a moderate decline and place it in front of a low-pulley cable with a rope attachment. Sit squarely on it, feet secured under the ankle pads. Lie back on the bench and grasp the ends of the rope with your hands at the sides of your head. Contract your abs to curl your body just short of perpendicular to the floor; avoid pulling through your hip flexors. Round your back as you rise; this increases the abdominal contraction. Lower yourself under control back to the start position.

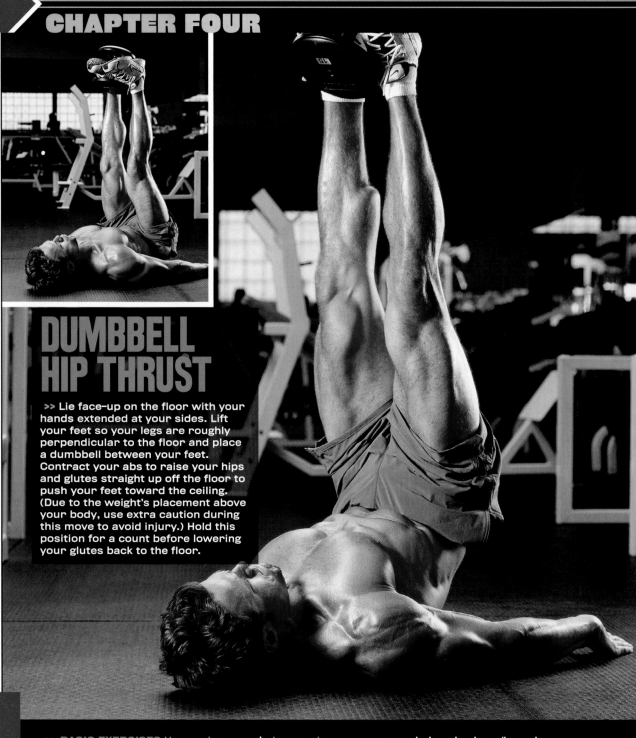

DUMBBELL HIP THRUST

>> Lie face-up on the floor with your hands extended at your sides. Lift your feet so your legs are roughly perpendicular to the floor and place a dumbbell between your feet. Contract your abs to raise your hips and glutes straight up off the floor to push your feet toward the ceiling. (Due to the weight's placement above your body, use extra caution during this move to avoid injury.) Hold this position for a count before lowering your glutes back to the floor.

>> **BASIC EXERCISES** Upper abs: **crunch;** Lower abs: **reverse crunch, hanging knee/leg raise**
>> **ADVANCED EXERCISES** Upper abs: **weighted crunch, machine crunch, decline bench cable crunch, kneeling cable crunch;** Lower abs: **exercise-ball pull-in, dumbbell hip thrust, weighted hanging leg raise;** Upper and lower: **double crunch**

WEIGHTED HANGING KNEE RAISE

>> Perform this exercise either hanging from a high bar (using straps is always an option) or on a vertical bench that supports your forearms. Hang at arm's length using an overhand grip, bending your knees 90 degrees and locking them in this position for the entire set. Hold a medicine ball between your knees or ankles. Without swinging your body, contract your abs to bring your knees toward your chest (at least above parallel to the floor) and lower under control, coming to a complete stop at the bottom so as not to generate momentum as you go into the next rep.

#98 YOUR NEXT AB WORKOUT

>>The following sample routine hits all areas of the midsection.

EXERCISE	SETS	REPS
Weighted Hanging Knee Raise or Dumbbell Hip Thrust	2-3	12-15
Decline Bench Cable Crunch	2-3	8-12
Decline Cable Twist	2-3	8-12
Weighted Plank	3	to failure*

* Between sets, rest as long as the previous set lasted.

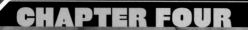

REGIONS 2 & 3
INTERNAL & EXTERNAL OBLIQUES

>> The obliques are off to either side of the rectus abdominis and run diagonally from your lower ribs to near your hipbone. The external obliques are the ones you can see, as they're superficial to the internal obliques, which are hidden underneath. The internal and external fibers run in opposite directions. Both the internal and external obliques are responsible for torso rotation and lateral flexion of the torso.

DECLINE CABLE TWIST

>> Place a decline bench in front of a cable stack with a D-handle attached to the low-pulley cable. Sit on the bench in a half sit-up position (your lower back shouldn't touch down) and hold the D-handle with both hands out in front of you. With your arms locked in that position, rotate your torso to the right until your right forearm is about parallel to the floor. Pause for a moment, return to the start, then repeat to the left side. That's one rep.

>> **BASIC EXERCISES** Lying crossover crunch, oblique crunch, jackknife
>> **ADVANCED EXERCISES** Oblique crunch on back extension bench, standing oblique cable crunch, decline cable Russian twist

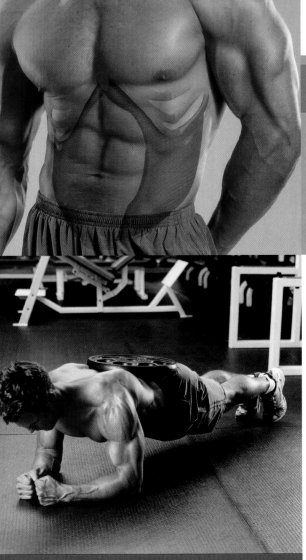

REGION 4
TRANSVERSE ABDOMINIS

>> The transverse abdominis lies beneath the rectus abdominis, and whereas the rectus fibers run vertically, the transverse fibers run horizontally. The main function of the transverse abdominis is initiating abdominal compression during an intense exhale. You'll find this function very useful during core exercises such as the plank, where you need to keep your navel drawn in tight, as well as in moves such as the woodchop and Russian twist.

ABSolutely GREAT TIPS

>> **FREQUENCY:** Abs can be trained from 3–5 days per week, depending on the load you place on them from one workout to the next. A session with weighted ab moves might require more days of rest afterward for recovery than one using strictly bodyweight exercises.

>> **VOLUME:** Vary the number of sets you perform, depending on how many times per week you train abs. If you train them twice a week, do four sets per exercise; if it's 4–5 times a week, do just two sets per exercise.

>> **SELECTION:** Choose four exercises for every ab training session — one each for the upper abs, lower abs, obliques and transverse abdominis.

>> **TIMING:** Begin your ab training with your weakest link. For most of us, that's the lower abs. If this is your weakest area, do exercises such as reverse crunches before moving on to exercises for your stronger areas. If obliques are your weakness, do oblique crunches first.

>> **LOAD/REPS:** Use varying degrees of resistance. Do weighted exercises to make your abs literally bigger and more pronounced, but also perform higher-rep/lighter-weight exercises that stress endurance. Unweighted sets should typically consist of 15–30 reps; weighted exercises can be performed in the 8–12 range, which is standard for muscle growth.

>> **WHEN:** Train abs after your weight session. Because the abs are so integral to stability and spinal safety, it's important not to fatigue them before a rigorous workout, especially on back or leg days.

WEIGHTED PLANK

>> Lie face-down on the floor with your body straight and arms extended in front of you. Have someone place a 25- to 45-pound plate on your lower back. Slowly lift your body off the floor onto your elbows and toes. Keep your abs pulled in tight and your back flat while holding this position for 30 seconds to begin with, then work toward longer periods.

>> **BASIC EXERCISES** Wood chop, lying leg raise >> **ADVANCED EXERCISES** Exercise-ball rollout, weighted plank

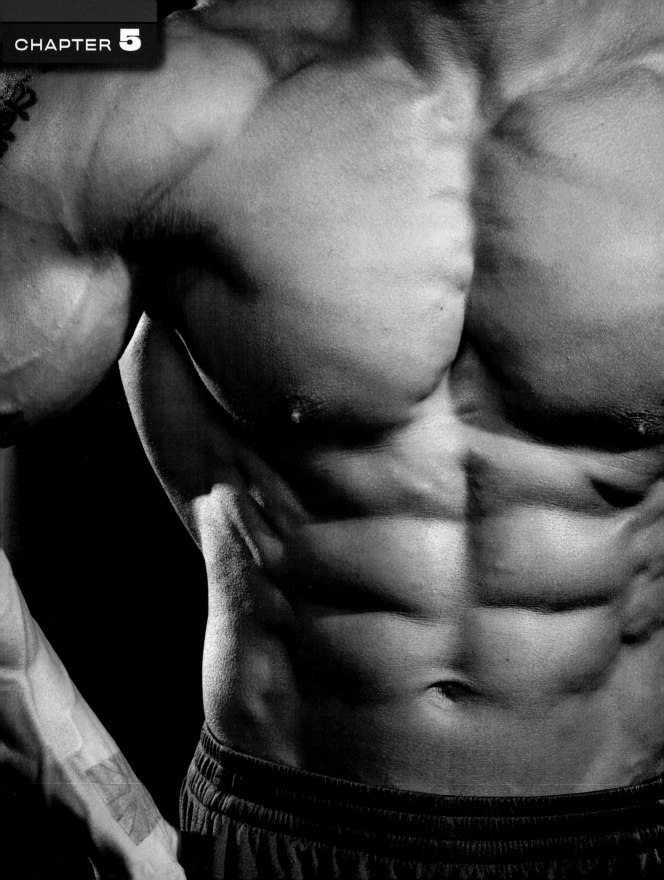

Better Abs In Five Weeks

Humans are creatures of habit, doing certain things over and over again because they feel comfortable, such as eating regularly at a favorite restaurant, driving the same route to work or doing the same exercise, set and rep schemes for a particular bodypart. Unfortunately, that last habit may be a big problem.

Getting into a rut with any muscle group isn't ideal, but it may be especially troublesome for abs. You don't need a PhD in exercise physiology to know that to make a muscle grow bigger and stronger you need to continually tax it with heavier loads or more repetitions, yet many of us often squeak by on a few sets of crunches tacked on to the end of a workout. Three sets, 20 reps each, rest and repeat.

This five-week program (outlined in chart form on page 96) solves both problems, breaking you out of a rut and introducing progression to your middle-management plan in the form of the weights you use, reps you complete and your rest periods between sets.

Well-defined abdominals don't happen by accident; it takes hard work and a carefully planned approach. Luckily for you, we've plotted out your sets, reps and exercises — all you need to add to see it through to the end are dedication and a bit of sweat equity.

SLAM-DUNK GUIDELINES

Our five-week plan requires you to train your midsection three times a week, resting at least 48 hours between sessions. If possible, do your ab work on days you're not training a major bodypart.

>> **Start by choosing one Group A exercise.** This group includes one move for each of the major regions of the abdominals — the upper abs, lower abs and obliques. Group A exercises add resistance to your bodyweight, meaning they are the most challenging moves in the workout and should be done early when you're fresh and high in energy. Since resistance levels can be manipulated one plate at a time, even beginner-level bodybuilders can perform these moves using a lighter weight.

Key to this exercise is choosing a weight with which you can perform only 10 reps; that will place the focus on building strength in your abominals. If you can't complete 10, the weight is too heavy; if you can do more than 10, the weight is too light. Be honest with yourself, because selecting the right resistance is critical to manipulating intensity during the program.

>> **Next, pick one move from Group B.** These intermediate-level exercises are slightly easier than Group A moves. Some Group B movements use added resistance — again, manipulate loads to fit your needs if you're a beginner.

Like Group A, this group has one exercise dedicated to lower abs, one for upper abs and one for obliques. Although you may want to alternate which area of

GROUP A STRENGTH BUILDERS

>> Choose one of these three Group A exercises, which are considered **advanced** moves because you can add resistance simply by changing the pin on the weight stack. Be sure to fine-tune the resistance so you hit the target rep (10) by adding/subtracting weight. For your ab workouts later that same week, choose one of the other moves each time. (Note: If you're not advanced, simply use a lighter resistance with which you can complete the recommended number of sets and reps.)

SETS + REPS | Do three sets of 10 reps the first week. Over the course of the next five weeks, add one plate (about 10 pounds) each week (so that by Week 5 you've added four plates), still trying to reach 10 reps but doing as many as you can.

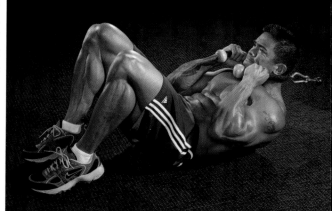

LYING CABLE CRUNCH
TARGET | Upper abs
Lie face-up directly in front of a low-pulley cable with a rope attached, with your knees bent and feet flat on the floor. Grasp the rope with a neutral grip, placing your hands by your ears and locking your arms in this position for the duration of the set. Contract your abs to curl up as high as you can, squeezing at the top, then lower yourself just enough so that your shoulder blades do not rest on the floor between reps.

PERFORMANCE POINTERS

1) Hold the peak contraction. If you consciously squeeze and momentarily hold the peak contraction at the top of each rep, you'll work your abdominals harder and be less inclined to race through your repetitions. Keep in mind, 10 slow and strict reps are better than 100 quick and sloppy ones.

2) Move at a smooth, deliberate pace. Use a slow, strict motion that increases the intensity of the contraction and minimizes momentum. Momentum is created using fast, explosive motions, which reduce workout quality and invite injury.

3) Exhale at the top of the move. Hold your breath until you've reached the peak-contracted position for a stronger, more intense contraction. Exhaling early reduces intra-abdominal pressure, so you won't be able to contract your abs as strongly.

4) Keep your head in line with your torso. When grasping your head to support it, don't interlock your fingers, which increases the likelihood you'll pull on your head and disrupt your spinal alignment. Lightly cup your fingers behind your head to support it — don't pull on it.

5) Make sure the action is restricted to your waist. During most upper and lower abdominal moves, your spine flexes (your lower back rounds), so don't keep your lower back arched during the movement. Keep other joints stabilized.

6) The range of motion is fairly small in many abdominal moves. Bringing your shoulder blades off the floor in the basic crunch, for example, works the abs through a full range of motion. Don't rise as high as you would in a full sit-up — such motion doesn't further contract or stimulate the abs and may increase hip flexor involvement when your feet are planted, as in decline-bench crunches.

7) Maintain constant tension throughout the set. Abs recover quickly, so if you rest between reps, even if for only a second, it becomes difficult to adequately fatigue the muscle.

8) Take precise rest periods between sets. After you complete your set, rest about 60 seconds to let your abs recover so you can complete your next set. If you start too early, they'll still be fatigued and you won't reach your target rep.

the abs you focus on as you progress through a workout, it's not required. In fact, one way to prevent the abdominals from becoming accustomed to a particular mode of training is to keep changing up the order of the moves.

The key with the second exercise is to choose a level of difficulty (via resistance or body position) that enables you to complete exactly 15 reps. The higher rep target works the abs in a slightly different way than that of the Group A exercise, building the ridges and valleys that make up a taut midsection. Hence, choosing the right resistance is an important factor in allowing you to achieve the target rep goal.

>> **Last, select a Group C exercise.** These are beginner-oriented bodyweight-only moves, but if you've been training hard thus far, they'll still be challenging. Again, there's one exercise for upper abs, one for lower abs and one for obliques, so the one you choose should be determined by which areas you've trained so far and what you want to focus on.

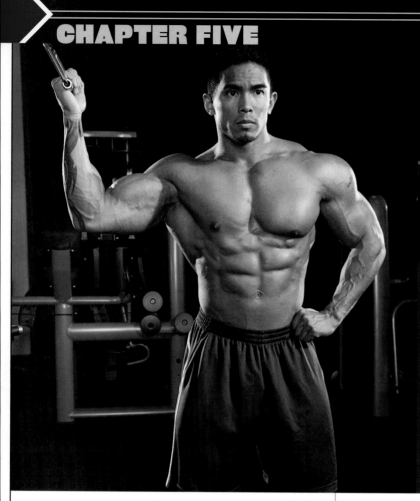

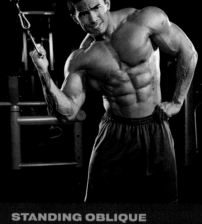

STANDING OBLIQUE CABLE CRUNCH

TARGET | Obliques

Stand about 2 feet away from a cable stack, your right shoulder facing the pulley. Attach a D-handle to the high cable and grasp it with an underhand grip, bending your arm about 90 degrees and locking it in this position for the duration of the set. Using your obliques, crunch down laterally as far as you can, holding the peak contraction briefly. Complete all reps for one side, then switch.

These moves turn up the fire even more by working in a higher rep zone. Aim for 20 reps per set; for people who find that goal too easy, we list ways to make them more difficult under each exercise description. At the higher rep range, your abs will feel the burn much sooner as you train them in a slightly different manner to emphasize muscle endurance.

>> **Rest periods for ab work vary by individual,** but start with a timed 60-second interval to determine if that's adequate. The abdominals are a fairly small muscle group that recovers quickly and doesn't require the same amount of rest between sets as larger bodyparts. You don't want your abs to recover fully before the next set.

>> **At your next ab-training session that week,** select an exercise from each group you did not perform in the previous training session(s). If you did the lower ab machine from Group A on Tuesday, pick one of the other two Group A movements on Thursday.

On your last abdominal training day that week, perform the remaining exercise. This strategy ensures that all areas of your abs get worked first when your energy levels are highest and through all the training zones: heavy for 10 reps to focus on strength, moderate for 15 reps to build size, and with bodyweight only for 20 reps to make the abs burn and build muscle endurance.

>> **Write it all down.** Keep a training log of the weights you used and exercises you selected; this will help you manipulate your training over the next five weeks.

THE NEXT LEVEL

We promised an ab workout that accounts for progression over time — that is, as your abs become stronger, you want to keep challenging them for continued progress. Here's how you'll do that in Week 2 and beyond:

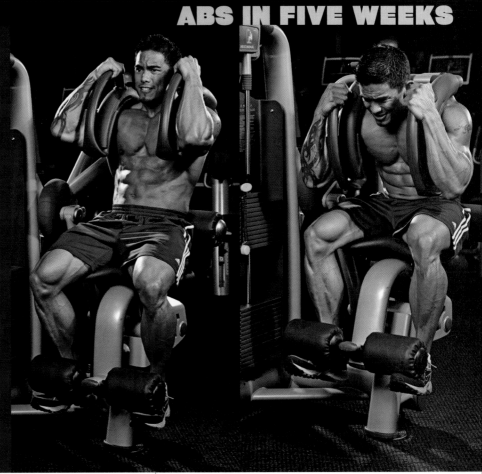

DOUBLE CRUNCH MACHINE

TARGET | Upper, lower abs

Sit inside the machine with your back flat against the pad. Hook your feet under the ankle pads and secure the shoulder pads firmly over your upper torso. Grasp the handles with both hands. With your head in a neutral position and eyes focused forward, crunch your upper body forward while simultaneously lifting your legs toward your upper body. Hold the peak contraction, then return to the start. Don't allow the weights to touch down between reps to keep constant tension on your abs.

>> **On all Group A moves, add one plate each week and still try for 10 reps per set.** Increasing the resistance in this progressive fashion makes the abs work harder. If you can't do 10 reps, no problem — the key is to increase the weight and complete as many reps as you can. This is why choosing the right weight in Week 1 is so important.

>> **On Group B moves, reduce the rest period between sets by five seconds each week.** During Week 2, rest just 55 seconds between sets. The third week, reduce the rest interval by another five seconds. Continue in this manner until you're resting only 40 seconds between sets by the fifth week. Progressively limiting your rest period is another way to increase workout intensity and make your abs stronger. You're still trying to reach the 15-rep target on every set for Group B exercises.

>> **On Group C moves, perform one additional rep each week,** keeping the resistance and rest intervals the same as in Week 1. In the second week, do 21 reps instead of 20, and increase that by one rep each week. By the fifth week, you're doing 24 reps for all sets of each Group C exercise.

DIAL IT IN

While the keys that drive this five-week abdominal program are variety and progression, it would be a mistake to think those two elements are all that's required to build washboard abs. Pay particular attention to your diet as well — monitoring carb and fat intake, total calories and following a smart supplementation program — while including at least four 30-minute cardio sessions a week to strip off bodyfat. Only through a potent combination of these elements can you truly carve a ripped six-pack.

At the end of five weeks, your abs will be much improved — and the proof will be in the mirror as well as in your advancing strength.

B SIZE BUILDERS

>> Choose one of these three Group B exercises, which are considered **intermediate** moves. Again, fine-tune the move to hit the target rep (15): for the decline-bench crunch, increase or decrease the angle of the bench; for the hanging knee raise, increase or decrease the bend in your knees; for the cable woodchop, add/subtract resistance. Select a different move for the week's second session, then do the remaining exercise in the final workout.

SETS + REPS | Perform three sets of 15 reps the first week. Over the course of the next five weeks, reduce your rest period between sets by five seconds each week (so by Week 3, you've cut 10 seconds off your rest period), still trying to do 15 reps each set. After five weeks, return to the normal rest period with which you can perform 15 reps — at this point, you should be able to do a more challenging variation of the move than when you started.

DECLINE-BENCH CRUNCH
TARGET | Upper abs
Set an adjustable bench to a moderate decline and sit squarely on it, with your feet secured under the ankle pads. Cup your hands lightly behind your head and lean backward. Contract your abs to curl up to a point just short of perpendicular to the floor; try to avoid pulling through your hip flexors. Round your back as you rise to increase the abdominal contraction, then lower under control.

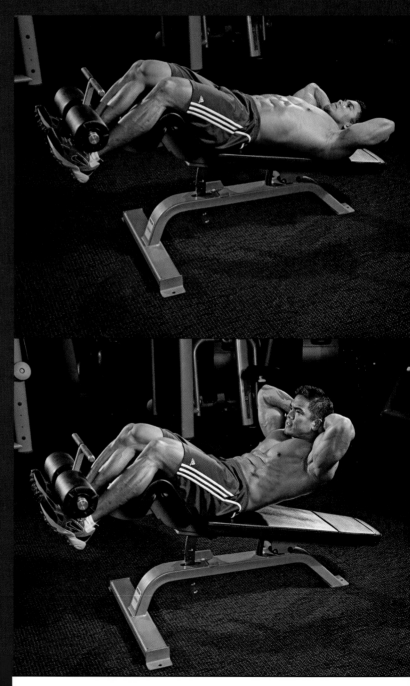

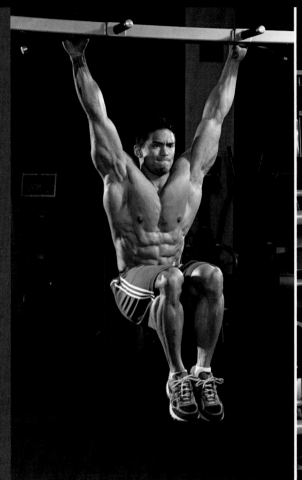

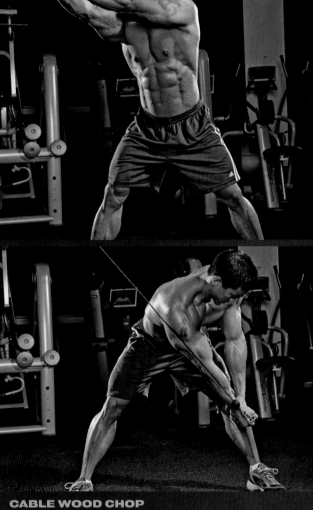

HANGING KNEE RAISE
TARGET | Lower abs

Perform this exercise either hanging from a high bar (using straps if you lose your grip before your abs fatigue) or on a vertical bench that supports your forearms. With an overhand grip, hang at arm's length, bending your knees 90 degrees and locking them in this position. Without swinging your body, contract your abs to bring your knees as high as you can into your chest and lower under control, coming to a stop at the bottom so you don't generate momentum before the next rep. Note: If you can easily hit the target rep, straighten your legs to make the move harder.

CABLE WOOD CHOP
TARGET | Upper abs, obliques

Stand erect with your feet outside shoulder width and knees slightly bent alongside a high-pulley cable (with a D-handle or I-handle attached), your right shoulder facing the pulley. Reach across your body with your left hand and grasp the handle, placing your right hand on top. Keep your arms straight but elbows unlocked throughout the set. Rotate your torso at the waist to the left by contracting your left obliques, pulling the handle down in an arc across your body to a position just below your knee. Keep your left arm as straight as possible. Return and repeat for reps. Do both sides.

The Five-Week
SIX-PACK SLAM

>> Select one exercise from each group, fine-tuning the resistance or your body position so you can just complete the targeted number of reps. For your next two workouts each week, choose an exercise not yet used. Follow this format throughout the five-week program.

#99 GROUP A: STRENGTH BUILDERS

CHOOSE ONE:	SETS	Week 1 REPS	Week 2 REPS	Week 3 REPS	Week 4 REPS	Week 5 REPS
Double Crunch Machine	3	10	up to 10	up to 10	up to 10	up to 10
Lying Cable Crunch	3	10	up to 10	up to 10	up to 10	up to 10
Standing Oblique Cable Crunch*	3	10	up to 10	up to 10	up to 10	up to 10

>> **INSTRUCTIONS** Week 1: Choose a resistance at which you can complete just 10 reps. Week 2: Add one plate to the weight used the previous week, trying to get the same number of reps (do as many as possible). Week 3: Add one more plate to what you used in Week 2. Week 4: Add another plate. Week 5: Add another plate.

#100 GROUP B: SIZE BUILDERS

CHOOSE ONE:	SETS	Week 1 REPS	Week 2 REPS	Week 3 REPS	Week 4 REPS	Week 5 REPS
Hanging Knee Raise	3	15	up to 15	up to 15	up to 15	up to 15
Decline-Bench Crunch	3	15	up to 15	up to 15	up to 15	up to 15
Cable Wood Chop*	3	15	up to 15	up to 15	up to 15	up to 15

>> **INSTRUCTIONS** Week 1: Choose a resistance or level of difficulty at which you can complete just 15 reps. Week 2: Reduce your rest period between sets by five seconds, aiming to do the same number of reps as the week before for all sets. Week 3: Reduce your between-sets rest period by another five seconds. Week 4: Remove another five seconds from your rest period. Week 5: Cut your rest period by five more seconds.

#101 GROUP C: ENDURANCE BUILDERS

CHOOSE ONE:	SETS	Week 1 REPS	Week 2 REPS	Week 3 REPS	Week 4 REPS	Week 5 REPS
Reverse Crunch	3	20	21	22	23	24
Supported Crunch	3	20	21	22	23	24
Oblique Crunch*	3	20	21	22	23	24

>> **INSTRUCTIONS** Week 1: Choose a variation of this bodyweight move that allows you to perform just 20 reps. Week 2: Do one additional rep on all sets using normal rest periods and the same resistance you used in Week 1. Week 3: Add another rep to all sets. Week 4: Do one more rep on all your sets. Week 5: Add another rep to all sets.

* Oblique movements require you to work each side individually.

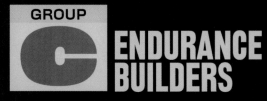

GROUP

ENDURANCE BUILDERS

>> Select one of these three Group C exercises, which are considered **beginner** moves done with just your bodyweight. Again, make slight adjustments in how you perform each exercise to fine-tune the degree of difficulty so you hit the target rep. For your next two ab sessions that week, choose one of the other moves each time.

SETS + REPS | Do three sets of 20 reps the first week. Over the course of the next five weeks, strive to do one more repetition per set each week, so that after five weeks you do 24 reps on each set (keeping the resistance and the rest periods unchanged). After five weeks, increase the level of difficulty of each move as you start again at 20 reps per set.

EXERCISE NOT SHOWN:

REVERSE CRUNCH
TARGET | Lower abs
This exercise can be found in Chapter 1, on page 53. In this particular program, you can also perform the reverse crunch on an incline board if you're more advanced and want to add an extra level of difficulty.

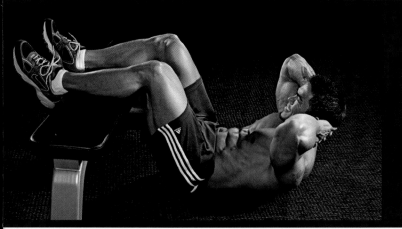

SUPPORTED CRUNCH
TARGET | Upper abs
Lie face-up on the floor with your heels up on a flat bench, hips and knees bent about 90 degrees. Cup your head lightly with your hands. Contract your abs to rise as high as you can, bringing your shoulder blades off the floor without pulling on your head. Lower under control. Note: To increase the level of difficulty, don't allow your shoulder blades to touch down at the bottom of each rep.

OBLIQUE CRUNCH
TARGET | Obliques
Lie on your left side, legs stacked with your knees bent, using your right hand to cup your head. Crunch up as high as you can, keeping the move in the lateral plane as much as possible to emphasize the obliques, and lower under control. Note: To increase the level of difficulty, simultaneously raise your feet a few inches off the floor.

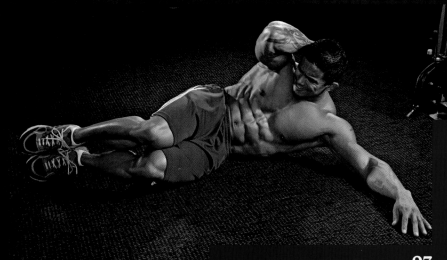

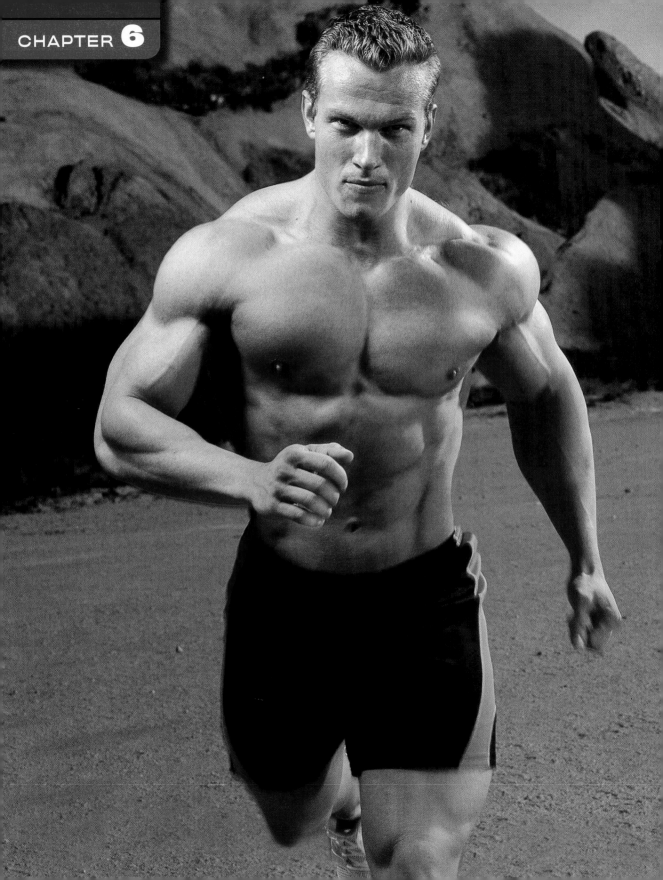

Complete Guide To Cardio

Sure, it's more fun to pick up a barbell and do a muscle-pumping set of biceps curls than jog mile after mile on a treadmill. With the barbell, you get instant gratification as your biceps swell with blood and get tight and pumped. Not so with cardio — heck knows running would be a lot more invigorating if you could actually watch the flab melt from your midsection with each step!

Cardio taps into your body's fat stores, shifts your calorie balance, improves your health and leaves you looking better for it. Knowing that uncovering the muscular, striated and vascular physique you're lifting weights for day after day requires aerobic activity, it's time to learn the basics.

First, some good news — you don't have to spend hours a day doing cardio. It doesn't have to be excruciating, and it definitely shouldn't feel like a chore. With that in mind, here are a few important guidelines that'll maximize your results.

CARDIO CONUNDRUM

Heading into the cardio section of the gym amounts to the fitness walk of shame for most gym rats. Not only do you *not* want to be there, but the seemingly endless aisles of baffling machines can be even more discouraging. You're there to nuke fat and would love it if someone could just tell you which machine will help you do that best. Allow us to do that for you.

Although little research compares the fat-burning effects of all the different cardio machines — treadmill, stationary cycle, stair-stepper, elliptical, etc. — there is research that compares the amount of fat burned on a treadmill vs. a stationary cycle. Scientists from the University of Birmingham (England) discovered that when male athletes exercised on a treadmill, they burned almost 30% more fat than when they used the stationary cycle at the same exercise intensities.

Although fat burned on other exercise equipment wasn't measured, you can reasonably assume that the same results would apply to other challenging upright exercises. An elliptical or cross-trainer machine, for example, involves the coordination of your lower body and upper body; thus, you consume more oxygen and burn more calories. If you avoid using the support rails on a stair-stepper or StepMill, you can achieve similar effects, along with an additional muscle-building — and calorie-burning — element.

So although a stationary cycle is still a viable option as a cardiovascular activity, you may want to choose a treadmill to burn the most fat; or hop on an elliptical, cross-trainer, StepMill or stair-stepper for similar results.

Here, we present five different programs, one of which will meet your fat-burning needs. Cardio has likely been working you over for years; now get ready to make it work *for* you.

THE BEST TIME TO BURN

Not sure when to perform your cardio for the greatest burn? Two times of day are best for doing cardio: the morning and after weights. In the morning, your body is in fat-burning mode due to your overnight fast. Cardio at this time of day on an almost empty stomach (see "Big Burn Nutrition" on the next page) also helps to regulate your circadian rhythm (internal clock), aiding sleep and recovery, and helping you to handle stress and feel better overall.

Doing cardio right after weight training, instead of before, allows you to hit the weights harder when your energy levels are highest and leads to three times higher growth hormone levels than when you do cardio first, scientists recently discovered.

It can also help you spot-reduce bodyfat from the areas you trained. A recent study from the University of Copenhagen (Denmark) found that subjects who did one-leg extensions significantly increased blood flow and fat release from the fat cells under the skin of the trained thigh compared to the resting thigh. That means when you lift weights, you free up fat from those areas, and if you immediately follow up with cardio, that freed-up fat gets burned for fuel and not redeposited on your body.

CARDIO KNOW-HOW

If you're going to do cardio, you want to make it worth your while. Keep these nine important tips in mind to maximize the amount of fat you burn (and the amount of muscle mass you maintain) during your sessions.

1) If nothing else, perform a bare minimum of 30 minutes of cardio at least three times per week to help keep your body in tune.

2) If a single, continuous session of cardio seems too boring, you can definitely break it up into shorter segments and still see results.

3) Do cardio either first thing in the morning or immediately after weightlifting. If neither of those times are possible in your schedule, just do it when you can — after all, that's certainly much better than not doing it at all.

4) Despite the abundance of technological advances

and new machines that have proliferated in gyms nationwide, the best cardio machine for fat-burning appears to be the good old treadmill.

5) Based on research, the best form of cardio for maintaining or enhancing leg mass and strength appears to be the stationary bike.

6) Working out at 70%–80% of your maximum heart rate (MHR) burns the most amount of fat during a cardio-focused workout session.

7) Interval training keeps your resting metabolism elevated higher after workouts, and may even lead to greater overall decreases in bodyfat over time, making it a solid option over a steady diet of "steady-state" cardio programming.

8) Eat 10–20 grams of protein or 3–6 grams of amino acids before cardio to preserve muscle.

9) Supplements such as caffeine, carnitine and hydroxycitrate (HCA) can help you burn more fat during cardio.

BIG BURN NUTRITION

Before cardio, stay away from certain foods like fats and, especially, carbs. Numerous studies show that eating carbs reduces the amount of fat burned during cardio, and eating fat before exercise has been shown to limit blood flow to exercising muscles.

So what should you eat? Take in a small amount of protein or amino acids before cardio workouts to prevent muscle breakdown; training on an empty stomach will force your body to turn to muscle as well as fat for fuel.

Ingesting whey protein or amino acids provides an alternative fuel and spares your muscles. One study from Japan found that when subjects consumed 3 grams of an amino-acid mixture before cardio, they burned more fat than those who took a placebo drink. Also consider other supplements that research shows will further enhance fat-burning during cardio, such as caffeine, carnitine and HCA.

STEADY BURN

Regardless of the cardio machine you choose, use the same exercise intensity to maximize the amount of fat burned. Research shows that on a treadmill or stationary bike, maximal fat-burning occurs at intensities about 70%–80% of your maximum heart rate (MHR = 220 – your age).

A 20-year-old, for example, has an MHR of 200 (220 – 20 = 200) beats per minute (bpm). Seventy percent of that would be 140 bpm (200 x 0.70). The most accurate measurements can be taken by palpating your radial pulse (thumb side of wrist) or carotid pulse (on side of neck under your jaw) for six seconds and multiplying the beats by 10.

Can't get it that way? Try the talk test. Research from the University of Wisconsin (La Crosse) discovered that the point where it started to become difficult for subjects to talk corresponded to 75%–80% of their MHR, the perfect range in which to burn fat. Work out at an intensity just below the point where it starts to become difficult to talk and you'll be burning bodyfat at a maximal rate. Try this workout — which has you exercising for the majority of time at 75% of your max heart rate — on a treadmill.

>> Try this targeted heart-rate workout on a treadmill or, if necessary, an elliptical machine, stair-stepper or stationary cycle. Adjust the machine so that you hit the prescribed intensities for the given intervals, which accommodate warming up and cooling down.

INTENSITY (% MHR)	TIME
50%	1 min.
60%	2 min.
75%	24 min.
60%	2 min.
50%	1 min.

BUILT TO LOSE

Balancing cardio with weight training is a constant struggle: You want to do cardio to get lean, but not at the expense of losing muscle. While diet, exercise intensity and a number of other factors will come into play, there is one choice you can make that will help your cause.

The key may be to focus on stationary cycling as your primary form of cardio. Scientists from the University of Jyväskylä (Finland) found that athletes who strength-trained and used a stationary cycle for 60 minutes twice per week gained more leg strength and thigh muscle size than those who just strength-trained. To keep the gains coming and the fat away, try this program three times a week, and be sure to keep your total cardio time to less than two hours per week.

>> Try this workout on a stationary cycle (upright or recumbent) three times per week to keep up the muscle gains and fat loss.

INTENSITY (% MHR)	TIME
50%	1 min.
60%	1 min.
70%	5 min.
75%	15 min.
70%	5 min.
60%	2 min.
50%	1 min.

INTERVAL CHALLENGE

Although training at 70%–80% of your MHR maximizes the amount of fat burned, it may not be the best way to maximize fat loss. Interval training — frequently alternating periods of high-intensity (80%–90% MHR) and low-intensity (50%–60% MHR) exercise — helped subjects lose the most body fat over a 20-week program, even though they burned more calories during steady exercise at a moderate intensity.

Why? High-intensity bouts keep your metabolism elevated at a higher rate and for a longer period after the exercise is over.

>> Try this 30-minute workout on a treadmill or other cardio station.

INTENSITY (% MHR)	TIME
50%	2 min.
60%	1 min.
80%	1 min.
50%	1 min.
85%	1 min.
50%	1 min.
90%	1 min.
50%	1 min.
90%	1 min.
50%	1 min.
90%	1 min.
50%	1 min.
90%	1 min.
50%	1 min.
90%	1 min.
50%	1 min.
90%	1 min.
50%	1 min.
90%	1 min.
50%	1 min.
90%	1 min.
50%	1 min.
90%	1 min.
50%	1 min.
90%	1 min.
50%	1 min.
85%	1 min.
50%	1 min.
80%	1 min.
50%	2 min.

Note: You don't have to measure your heart rate every minute to figure out your intensity. Once you know the treadmill speed that gets your heart rate to the desired level, adjust the workout each minute by speed.

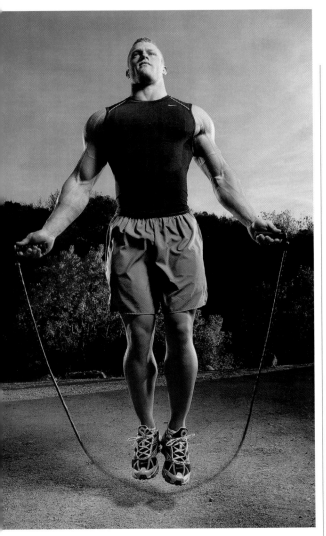

subjects performed three 10-minute bouts of running on a treadmill (about 80% MHR) separated by 20-minute rest periods, they burned the same amount of calories and fat as when they did one 30-minute run at the same intensity. Try the workout given here, separating each 10-minute session with a bodypart workout. For example, on chest, triceps and abs day, train chest and then do cardio, triceps then cardio, and abs then cardio.

>> To minimize boredom and still burn fat, do this workout three times in a day on your choice of cardio machines. You could even alternate machines for each of the three bouts.

INTENSITY (% MHR)	TIME
50%	1 min.
60%	1 min.
75%	6 min.
60%	1 min.
50%	1 min.

PYRAMID

Doing cardio at a steady state for long periods can get boring, so if you want to mix up your intensity, one way to do so is to train at a high intensity for half the workout and then use a low intensity for the other half, with the tougher portion coming first.

Scientists recently reported that when subjects exercised on a stationary cycle at 80% MHR for the first 15 minutes and finished the final 15 minutes at a more leisurely 60% MHR, they burned 25% more fat than when they reversed the order of intensity. Try the workout below to keep boredom (and fat) at bay.

>> Try this pyramid-intensity workout on a treadmill or stationary cycle to burn 25% more fat.

INTENSITY (% MHR)	TIME
50%	1 min.
60%	1 min.
80%	15 min.
60%	15 min.
50%	1 min.

BOREDOM BUSTER

You can't sit through an entire TiVo'd episode of *Lost*, much less a nonstop 30-minute cardio bout? Not to worry. Your total time spent doing cardio exercise is what's important for burning more calories and fat.

If cardio bores the hell out of you, you should still try to get the prescribed minimum of 30 minutes three times a week. But that doesn't mean the half-hour of cardio has to be continuous — you can break it up into 10-minute sessions and still burn the same amount of fat. Scientists from the University of Missouri (Columbia) found that when male and female test

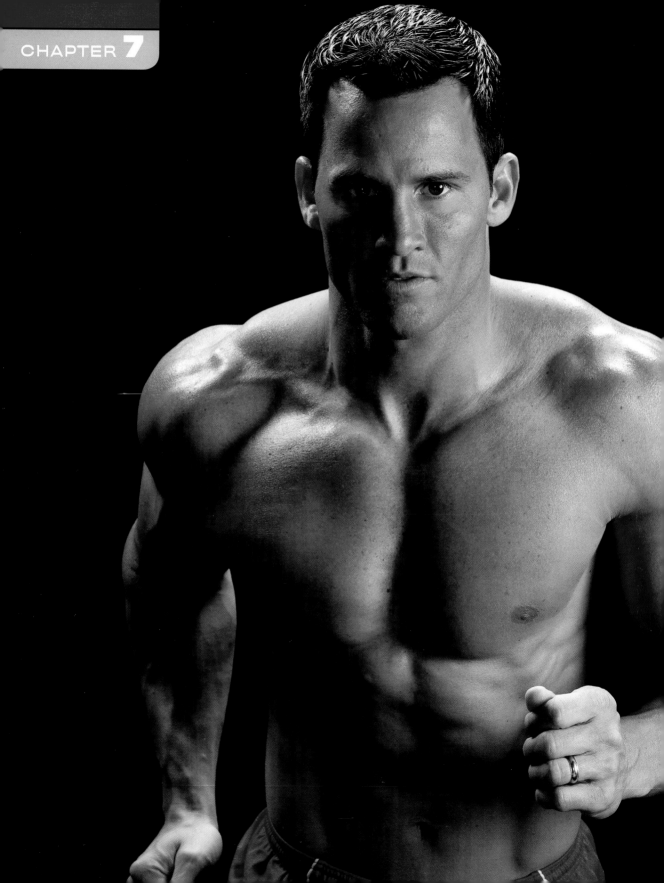

Fit With HIIT

Less is more...except when it applies to things you don't necessarily enjoy, that is. Take cardio, for example. How much cardio does it take to burn through that stubborn layer of fat lingering around your abdomen? If you've believed the prevailing opinions of exercise experts over the years, copious amounts — or at least that's what it feels like at times, since the most pervasive methodology behind fat-burning involves seemingly interminable sessions of cardiovascular activity done at a sustained rate. Where cardio is concerned, the theory has always been more is more.

But all that's about to change. What would you say if we told you that the latest scientific research suggests shorter cardio sessions for increased fat loss? How would you feel if you could actually end up burning more fat in the long run while holding on to more of your muscle? You can go ahead and smile — because it's entirely true. High-intensity interval training, or HIIT, is on the fast track to becoming the standard for steady and sustained fat loss. Turn the page and start learning more about this exciting breakthrough.

CHAPTER SEVEN

THE HIIT LIST

Here are three sample HIIT workouts. The training modes listed are examples; feel free to substitute other cardio choices. Each sprint, whether on foot or a stationary cycle, indicates an all-out effort. Perform the active recovery intervals at a slow-enough pace to prepare you for the next sprint.

TREADMILL SPRINT

Intensity	Time	Elevation
Warm-up	2–3 min.	0
Walk	1 min.	0
Sprint	1 min.	1
Walk	1 min.	0
Sprint	1 min.	1
Walk	1 min.	0
Sprint	1 min.	1
Walk	1 min.	0
Sprint	1 min.	3
Walk	1 min.	0
Sprint	1 min.	5
Walk	1 min.	0
Sprint	1 min.	5
Walk	1 min.	0
Sprint	1 min.	5
Walk	1 min.	0
Sprint	1 min.	5
Walk	1 min.	0
Sprint	1 min.	5
Walk	1 min.	0
Sprint	1 min.	5
Walk	1 min.	0
Sprint	1 min.	5
Walk	1 min.	0
Sprint	1 min.	5
Cool-down	2–3 min.	0

TOTAL: 28–30 MINUTES

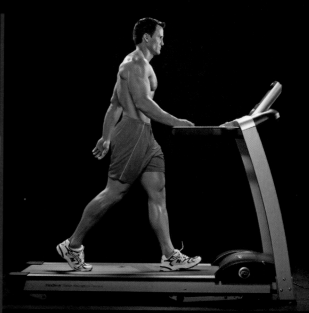

TIP: Consider the time it takes the treadmill to reach your incline and sprint speed by adjusting 5–10 seconds early.

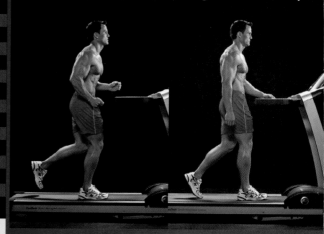

OUTDOOR SPRINT

Intensity	Time
Warm-up	2–3 min.
Sprint	10 sec.
Slow walk	20 sec.
Sprint	10 sec.
Slow walk	20 sec.
Sprint	10 sec.
Slow walk	20 sec.
Sprint	10 sec.
Slow walk	20 sec.
Perform circuit seven times for 14 minutes total	
Slow walk	2–3 min.

TOTAL: 18–20 MINUTES

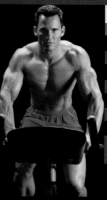

STATIONARY BIKE

Intensity	Time
Warm-up	2–3 min.
Sprint	30 sec.
Slow pedal	30 sec.
Sprint	30 sec.
Slow pedal	30 sec.
Sprint	30 sec.
Slow pedal	30 sec.
Perform circuit eight times for 24 minutes total	
Cool-down	2–3 min.

TOTAL: 28–30 MINUTES

With HIIT, the workouts are shorter, yes, but you'll actually be working harder than the guy on the treadmill next to you. HIIT is what it says — high-intensity — and the results are undeniable. If you're used to wearing a heart-rate monitor to judge the efficiency of your cardio, shelve it — you won't need it. By cycling between bouts of all-out effort and short stretches of active recovery, a mirror will be all you need to gauge your progress.

BURNING DEBATE

Bodybuilders and others have long used steady-state cardio, which involves low- to moderate-intensity exercise performed at 60%–70% of one's maximum heart rate (MHR), to whittle away bodyfat. Trainers and other experts argue that since lower-intensity cardio exercise burns a higher percentage of fat for energy, slow and steady indeed wins the race.

HIIT cardio, on the other hand, involves intervals of high-intensity exercise — at a rate near 90% MHR — followed by intervals of slower-paced active recovery. Anecdotal reports and early research on HIIT went against the steady-state establishment, claiming that it was the superior method of cardio for losing fat. And the exercise community, likely looking for a way to collectively limit its time on a conveyor belt, felt it was time for in-depth science to put an end to the developing debate. What they found, time after time, was that HIIT cardio was the best way to lose fat, despite the fact that it required less total time.

One of the earliest studies, done by researchers at Laval University (Ste-Foy, Quebec, Canada), kept it basic, using two groups in a months-long experiment. One group followed a 15-week program using HIIT, while the other performed only steady-state cardio for 20 weeks. Proponents of steady-state training were pleased to hear that those subjects burned 15,000 calories more than their HIIT counterparts. Those who followed the HIIT program, however, lost significantly more bodyfat.

A 2001 study from East Tennessee State University (Johnson City) demonstrated similar findings with subjects who followed an eight-week HIIT program. Again, HIIT proved to be the better fat-burner — subjects dropped 2% bodyfat over the course of the experiment. Meanwhile, those who plodded through the eight weeks on a steady-state program lost no bodyfat.

The most recent study, out of Australia, reported that a group of females who followed a 20-minute HIIT program consisting of eight-second sprints followed by 12 seconds of rest lost an amazing six times more bodyfat than a group that followed a 40-minute cardio program performed at a constant intensity of 60% MHR.

TURN UP THE HIIT

So what is it about HIIT cardio training that sends bodyfat to the great beyond? There are actually several explanations, but the first and perhaps most important involves its effect on metabolism.

A 1996 study from Baylor College of Medicine (Houston) reported that subjects who performed a HIIT workout on a stationary cycle burned significantly more calories during the 24 hours following the workout than those who cycled at a moderate, steady-state intensity. Why? Since HIIT is tougher on the body, it requires more energy (calories) to repair itself afterward. That means a rise in resting metabolism.

The previously mentioned 2001 East Tennessee State study found that test subjects in the HIIT program also burned nearly 100 more calories per day during the 24 hours after exercise. More recently, a study presented by Florida State University (Tallahassee) researchers at the 2007 Annual Meeting of the American College of Sports Medicine reported that subjects who performed HIIT cardio burned almost 10% more calories during the 24 hours following exercise than a steady-state group, despite the fact that the total calories burned during each workout were the same for both groups.

Research also confirms that HIIT enhances the metabolic machinery in muscle cells that promotes fat-

CHAPTER SEVEN

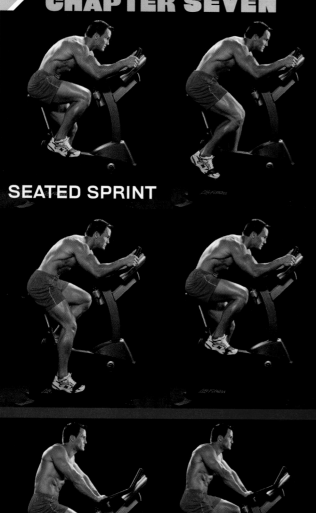

SEATED SPRINT

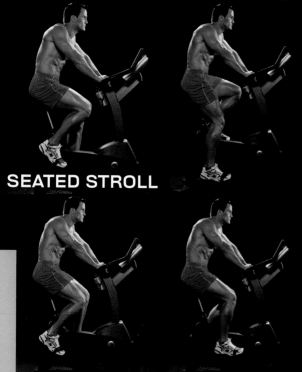

SEATED STROLL

MAXIMIZING FAT-BURNING

NOW THAT YOU KNOW WHICH CARDIO METHOD
WORKS BEST FOR MAXIMUM FAT LOSS, COMBINE
THESE TIPS WITH YOUR HIIT CARDIO TO SPEED
YOUR PROGRESS

>> Time your HIIT sessions Doing cardio after
weights or in the morning on an empty stomach
will burn the greatest amount of fat. During both of
these times your body is slightly carb-depleted,
making fat the primary fuel source for energy.

>> Preserve muscle If you do cardio first thing in
the morning, have a half-scoop of whey protein
(about 10 grams) mixed in water or 6–10 grams of
mixed amino acids before your session. This will
help ensure that your body draws most of its
energy from fat and these fast-digesting supplements instead of your muscle.

>> Supplement right A fat-burning stack of caffeine
and carnitine will enhance the amount of fat you
burn during exercise. Take 200–400 mg of caffeine
along with 1.5–3 grams of carnitine (in the form of
L-carnitine, acetyl-L-carnitine or L-carnitine
L-tartrate) 30 minutes before your session.

>> Make it an uphill climb Consider working hills
into your HIIT cardio to add more detail to your
hams and glutes. If you don't have hills available,
adjust the incline on a treadmill to simulate the
effect. Be sure to drop the incline to level, or zero,
during low-intensity intervals.

>> Get in and out If you limit HIIT cardio sessions to
20–30 minutes, you'll actually be aiding muscle
growth and preventing muscle loss.

>> Adjust for the lag During intervals on a treadmill, there will be a slight lag time as the machine
adjusts to the change in speed: By the time the
treadmill is up to running speed, the fast interval
portion is almost over. To keep your intensity high,
begin the sprint portion of the interval when the
machine has reached your target speed. You can
do this by counting seconds once the target speed
is reached, or by straddling the sides of the treadmill as it gets up to speed.

burning and blunts fat production. In the previously mentioned Laval University study, scientists noted that the HIIT subjects' muscle fibers had significantly higher markers for fat oxidation (fat-burning) than those in the steady-state exercise group. And a study published in a 2007 issue of the *Journal of Applied Physiology* reported that young females who performed seven HIIT workouts over a two-week period experienced a 30% increase in both fat oxidation and levels of muscle enzymes that enhance fat oxidation.

Moreover, researchers from the Norwegian University of Science and Technology (Trondheim) reported that subjects with metabolic syndrome — a combination of medical disorders that increases one's risk of cardiovascular disease and diabetes — who followed a 16-week HIIT program had a 100% greater decrease in the fat-producing enzyme fatty acid synthase compared to subjects who followed a program of continuous moderate-intensity exercise.

The bonus to all this research is discovering that shorter exercise sessions will allow you to hold on to more muscle. Pro physique competitors often have to walk a fine line between just enough and too much steady-state cardio because the usual prescription of 45–60 minutes, sometimes done twice a day precontest, can rob muscles of size and fullness. Short, hard bursts of cardio, on the other hand, will help you preserve your hard-earned muscle mass.

To illustrate the point, think about the typical size of a marathon runner's legs compared to a sprinter's legs. The sprinter — whose entire training schedule revolves around HIIT — possesses significantly more muscular thighs. In the event you choose cycling as your primary method of HIIT cardio, you can actually add leg mass because of the increased recruitment of the growth-crazy, fast-twitch fibers in your thigh musculature.

When considering all the science, you might just come to the conclusion that HIIT could be the *only* way to train for people looking to lose fat while adding and/or preserving muscle mass.

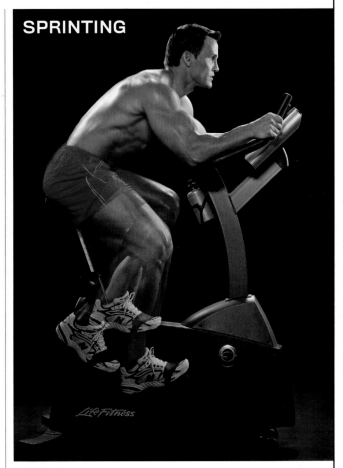

SPRINTING

REV IT UP

Cardio is a necessary component of reaching your physique goals. And now we know it doesn't need to be monotonous to be effective — this chapter has outlined the science to prove it.

Turning up the heat on your workouts with HIIT will keep your gym time productive while speeding up your fat oxidation — and in less time than you'd normally spend doing cardio. If steady-state is the four-door sedan of cardio, HIIT is the Porsche — it's sexier, and there's enough under the hood to keep you blowing past the guy next to you. Try it for yourself.

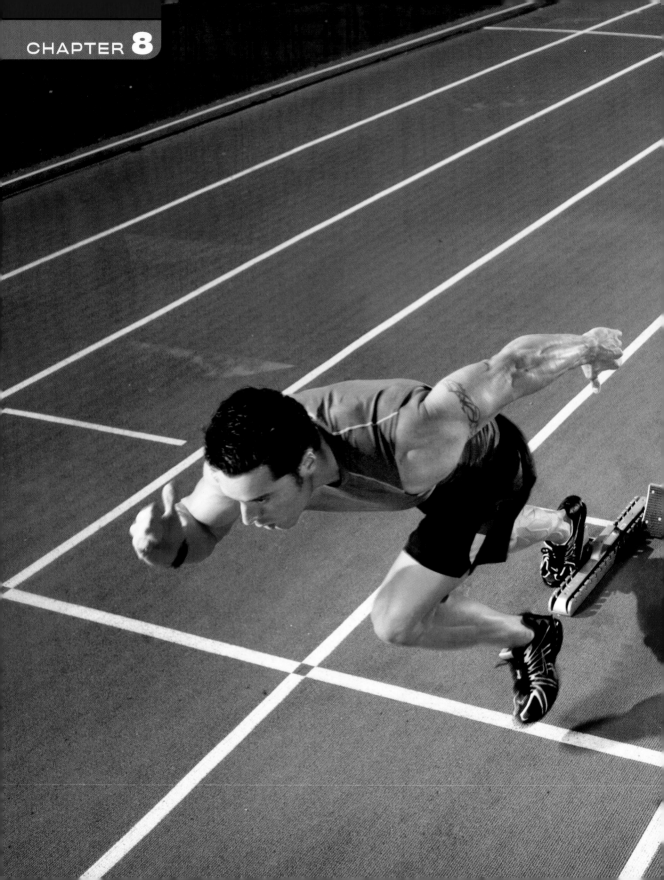

Sprint To A Leaner Physique

If a picture is worth a thousand words, then take a moment to search the web for photos of the world's top sprinters. Maurice Greene. Usain Bolt. Tyson Gay. Asafa Powell. More often than not, they've got muscle — and not just in their legs.

In fact, if there's one hallmark of the great sprinters of our time, it's their quarterhorselike physiques: densely muscled thighs propelling barrel-chested torsos down tracks at dangerously high speeds.

The equivalent doesn't really exist on the long-distance side of the equation. Envision a marathon runner and what do you come up with? A spindle-shanked Kenyan in short-shorts. Not quite the inspiration you're looking for as someone hoping to build a bigger, muscular body.

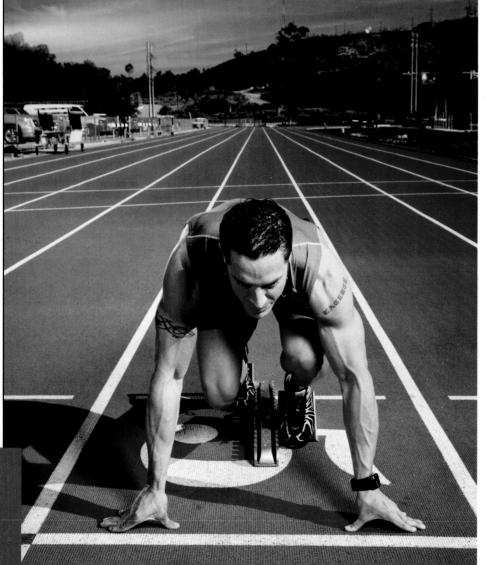

In Chapter 7, we told you about an indoor cardio program called HIIT, or high-intensity interval training. Based on the latest research regarding interval training routines, HIIT tapped the well of exercise science to show conclusively that short, lung-searing bouts of cardio are more effective at burning fat than longer, steady-pace turns on a treadmill or exercise bike. Among the chief benefits to test subjects was an increased resting metabolism over the subsequent 24 hours that resulted in a greater number of calories burned than their more languidly trained brethren. Although the overall calorie dump during exercise was higher for the steady-state subjects in one study's head-to-head comparisons, those on the HIIT program lost significantly more body-fat — and that's the objective here.

Before we bore you into fat gain by documenting all the research in favor of sprint work, let us be clear: Science is on the side of HIIT as the most efficient way to burn fat while preserving muscle mass. But you don't really need science to tell you that; the empirical reality of the benefits of sprint work has been blowing down red rubber tracks in front of our eyes for years.

ON TRACK

In the aforementioned chapter on HIIT training, we provided an

By taking your workouts out to a local track, you're in effect periodizing cardio to keep your body from getting used to the same old routines.

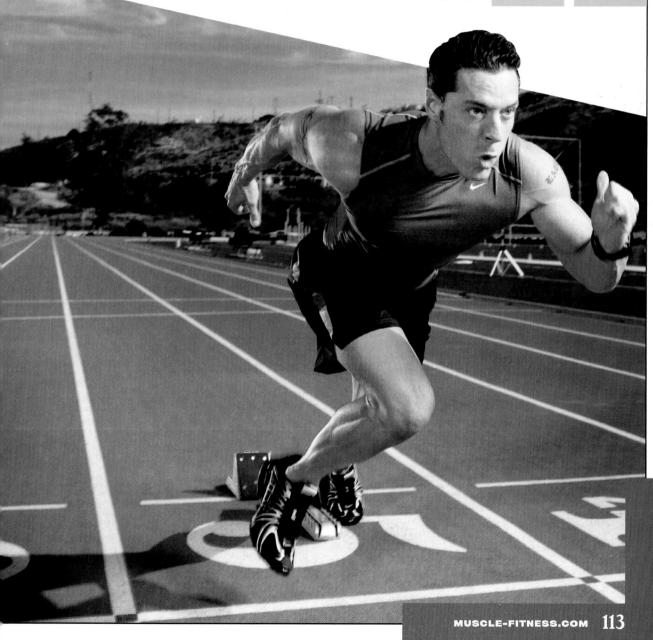

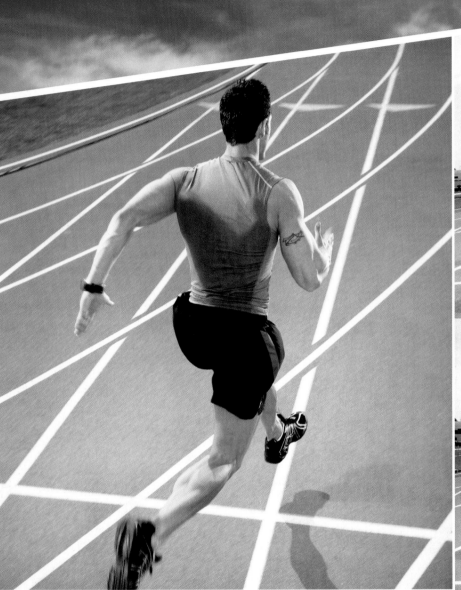

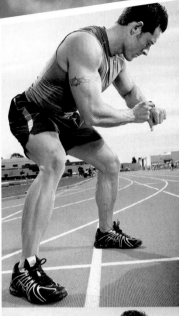

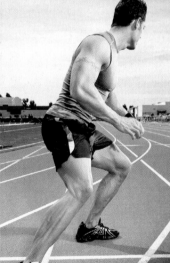

interval training program designed for treadmills and exercise bikes, partly because most of you do your cardio in the gym and partly because track work in the biting cold of winter appeals only to Russo-Siberians in Murmansk.

But by taking your workouts to a local track when the weather cooperates, you're in effect periodizing your cardio to keep your body from acclimating to the same old routines, and you're countering the desire to drop your cardio altogether. The advantages of the seven sprint workouts presented here are variety, adaptability and ease of use. You don't need a heart-rate monitor or even a personal trainer to push buttons for you. You need a track, a watch and some good shoes.

All you need for this program are shoes, a watch and a track.

Sprint Interval
INSTRUCTION

Some of the sprint intervals in this chapter aren't for the faint of heart. But with seven options, there's something for everyone, and the variety will keep your workouts from becoming tedious before their time. Where you see "sprint-to-stride" (in the 30-second and one-minute sprint intervals), maintain your pace for as long as possible, then, as you fatigue, slow down but keep pushing hard until the end.

Before each workout, take 5–10 minutes to warm up. Make sure you stretch appropriately so your muscles' range of motion is sufficient for the sprinting ahead. And, for the sake of convenience, do your best to find an actual track.

» 10-Second Sprint Training

TOTAL TIME 20 minutes

INTERVAL
10-second sprint + one-minute jog
Repeat for a total of 18 minutes
This is a continuous-motion interval. Do not stop between sprints: Ease into the one-minute jogs, then ramp back up into the sprints.

COOL-DOWN Walk for two minutes

» Brief & Brutal Sprint Program

TOTAL TIME 24–32 minutes

INTERVAL
30-second sprint-to-stride + one-minute walk
Repeat three times

COOL-DOWN Walk for two minutes
Repeat cycle 2–3 times

» The Minute Man

TOTAL TIME 32–48 minutes

INTERVAL
One-minute sprint-to-stride + two-minute walk
Repeat three times

COOL-DOWN Walk for four minutes
Repeat cycle 1–2 times

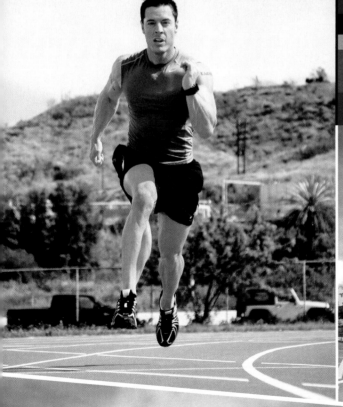

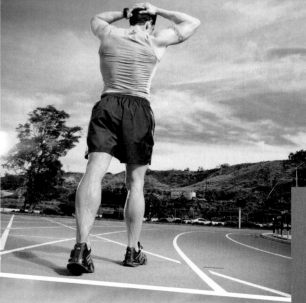

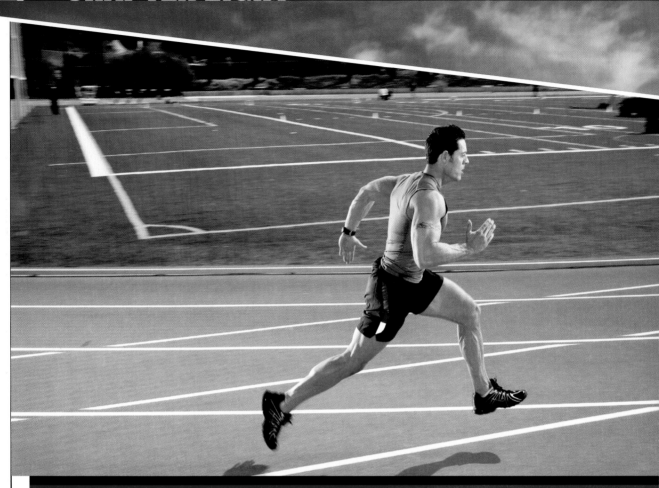

Sprint Interval **INSTRUCTION** (cont.)

» Out of the Blocks

TOTAL TIME 25–30 minutes

INTERVAL
40-yard sprint + walk back to start

COOL-DOWN Rest for two minutes after
each sprint as you walk back to the start
Complete 10 sprints total

» Up & Back Interval

TOTAL TIME 25–30 minutes

INTERVAL
Sprint 100 meters + walk back to start
Sprint 200 meters + walk back to start
Sprint 300 meters + walk back to start
Sprint 400 meters + walk back to start

COOL-DOWN Rest five minutes
Repeat cycle in reverse order

» 4x4 Interval

TOTAL TIME About 30 minutes

INTERVAL
100-meter sprint + walk 100 meters
Repeat three times

COOL-DOWN Rest for three minutes
Repeat cycle three times

» Seven the Hard Way

TOTAL TIME 25–35 minutes

INTERVAL
7 40-meter sprints + walk back to start
7 100-meter sprints + walk back to start

COOL-DOWN After each sprint, rest an additional
30 seconds beyond the time it takes to walk back, then
repeat
If you're up for an additional challenge: Instead of 40-
and 100-meter sprints, do 100- and 200-meter sprints

Some exercise experts still insist that steady, long-duration cardio (30–60 minutes) is the best way to get fit and lose fat, but we're here to tell you that shorter bouts of intense work can also reap benefits for you. Simply put, when faced with a small window in which to get your cardio done, you're better off speeding around a track a few times than strolling on a treadmill for an hour. In other words, short and intense is better than short and slow, or even long and slow.

Depending on your goals, use our programs 1–3 times per week, not every day, and use just one of the interval options per day. Some are shorter than 30 minutes, some longer, so choose according to your schedule.

We can't guarantee that you'll ever be mistaken for a wind-aided Usain Bolt, but we're certain nobody will confuse you with Robert Kipkoech Cheruiyot, either.

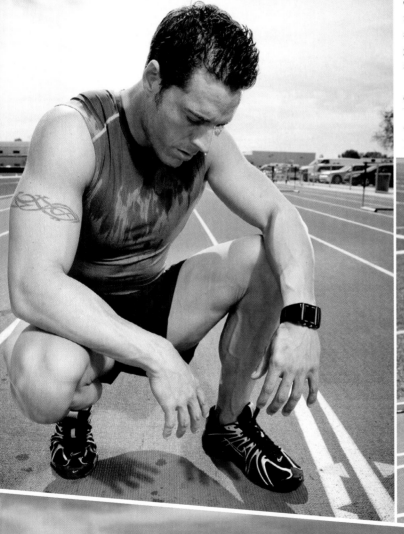

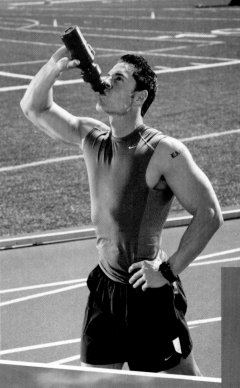

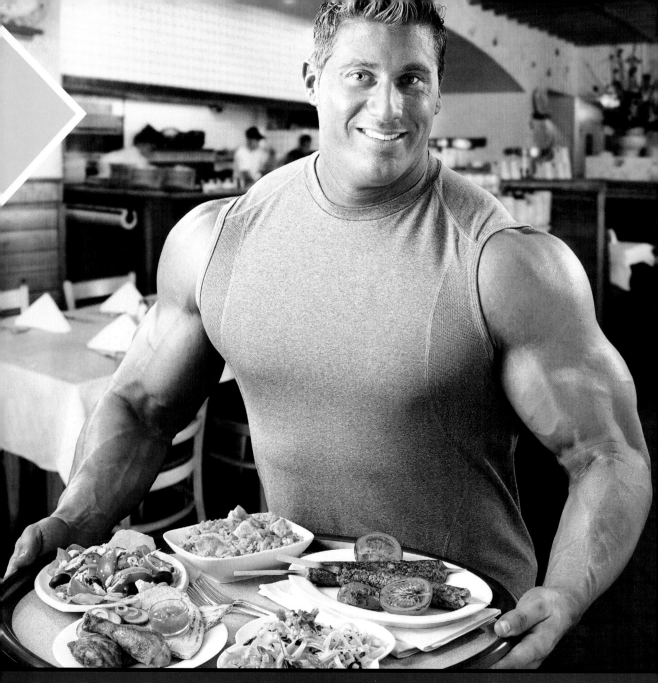

SECTION TWO
NUTRIT

An impressive physique is not built through weights and cardio alone. In fact, it's quite clear that diet and nutrition are the most important parts of the body-transforming equation. The following chapters provide you with healthy meal plans, expert advice and easy recipes to ensure that all of your hard training doesn't go to waste.

ION

 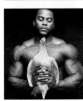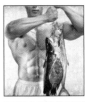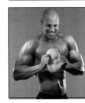
nutrition contents

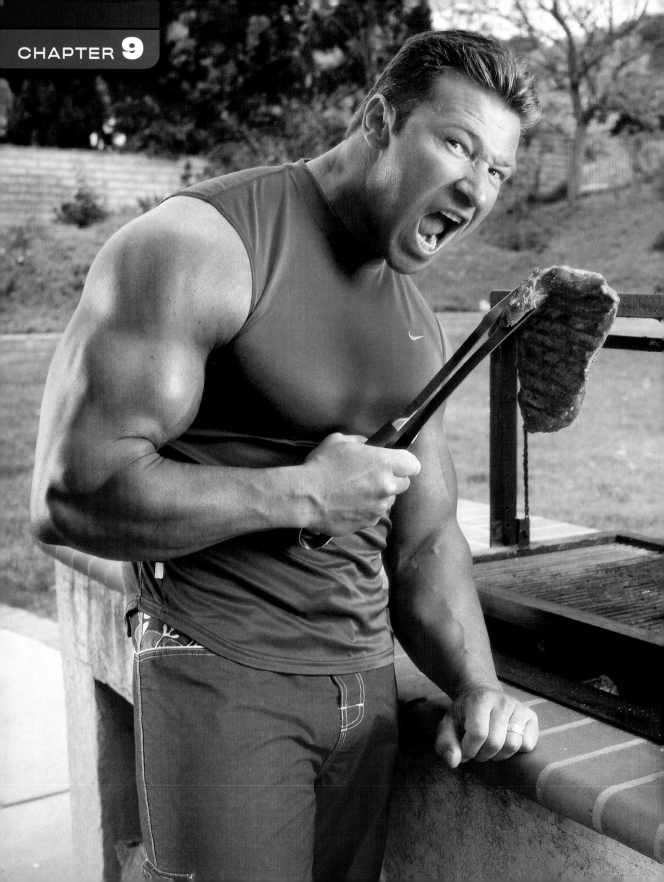

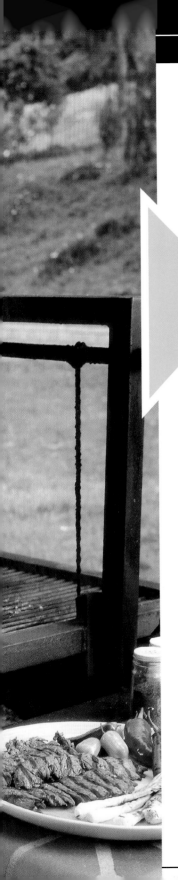

The Burn-Zone Diet

Do you have size, but not definition?
If you've been in mass-gain mode for a while, and you've packed on appreciable pounds — some muscle, some bodyfat — now may be the time to sculpt and refine your physique. With our help, you can do just that, and get great results in as little as 30 days.

Your first instinct may be to simply cut your carbohydrates to the bare-bones minimum. That approach could provide dividends, at least initially, but going without carbs for too long can slow your metabolism, which will set back your efforts and lead to frustration.

Your metabolism adapts to diets and exercise, so you have to know how and when to make changes on both of those fronts to achieve the desired effect. The following diet plan tackles this problem in three ways without slowing your metabolism: It creates a calorie deficit to ramp up your fat-burning ability; it incorporates specific cardio workouts to accelerate fat loss; and it includes certain supplements to keep the calorie-burning fire stoked.

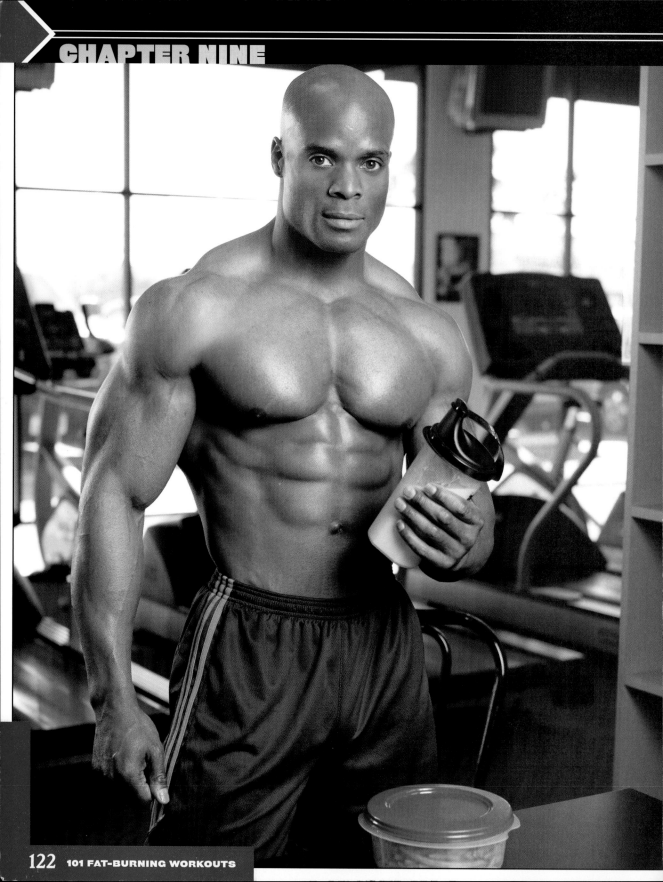

CALORIE CONUNDRUM

The major cutbacks in your food intake will focus specifically on carbohydrates and fat. In fact, this meal plan — built for five days, starting over on the sixth — eliminates most dietary fat and limits carbs to two servings per day. When the body senses this reduction, it calls on bodyfat stores to make up for the loss, thus helping to burn out the bad stuff. The complications ensue when you mess with your carb levels.

Full muscles come from eating this much-reviled macronutrient, which binds with water and lives in your muscles as "muscle glycogen." In general, the more carbs stored in your muscles, the bigger and, to a degree, harder they appear. This is why many top bodybuilders look very lean even when their bodyfat rises in off-season mass-gain mode. Their muscles are full of glycogen, creating an illusion of leanness.

When you want to *actually* get ripped, turning the illusion of leanness into a sinewy reality, you must eliminate the bulk of your dietary carbs because they interfere with the breakdown of bodyfat. So how do you keep your muscles full without carbs to feed them? By intermittently filling them with glycogen.

The first four days of this low-calorie, low-carb diet could make a monk shudder. But on the fifth day, higher calories and carbs are the keys to keeping both your muscles looking full and your metabolism firing. This day of higher carbohydrate intake can coax the body into believing that the diet phase is over, which may prevent your metabolism from slowing down. This carb ramp-up is vital to the entire process, not only for muscle fullness and metabolic rate, but for your energy levels, as well, which may lag during much of this program.

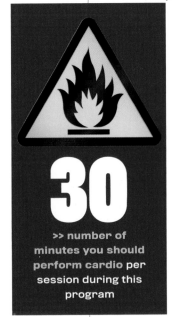

30

>> number of minutes you should perform cardio per session during this program

THE MEAL PLAN

The foundation of this diet, built for a 180-pound male but applicable to someone weighing 160–200 pounds, is four days (Meal Plan A) of restricted calories and carbs followed by a fifth day (Meal Plan B, which includes two options) that increases both to trick the body into believing the drought is over. Then you repeat the process.

For some of you, however, it won't be quite that simple. Since everyone responds differently to diets, you might have to make adjustments. For example, if by Day 4 you're looking really good, you can extend your time on Meal Plan A by another day before switching to Plan B on the sixth day, then repeating the process. On the other hand, if you're totally flat and tired by the third day using Meal Plan A, implement Plan B on Day 4, one day earlier than scheduled. Then start again from the beginning.

Remember: Every body responds differently to a diet. As a precaution against a possible metabolic meltdown, we recommend you take a handful of fat-burning supplements. First, consider taking 25–100 milligrams of active guggulsterones three times a day. This herb-based agent can prevent your thyroid hormones, which oversee your metabolic rate, from diving. Next, try 2–3 grams of carnitine before and after all workouts, especially cardio; carnitine facilitates fat-burning and prevents the breakdown of muscle tissue, which in turn protects your metabolism and may even support testosterone uptake by muscles. Finally, try some thermogenic agents. They can increase your levels of norepinephrine, a hormone that boosts metabolism and triggers fat-cell breakdown, increasing fat metabolism. Taken in the morning, before cardio and again before training, thermogenics can increase the number of calories the body burns each day. Since getting shredded is the goal, don't skip this step.

RUNNING MAN

The diet will make a difference in your physique, but cardio will help round out your results. First thing in the morning, before you eat, is a great time for aerobic activity. Since you've been fasting all night and haven't eaten carbs for a while, your blood sugar will be low. As a result, your body will dig into its bodyfat stores for energy. Or, if you prefer to keep your weight and cardio training together, do cardio right after weights.

Research shows that this can help you burn even more fat than when you do cardio first thing in the morning on an empty stomach.

On the intensity front, harder is always better. You can try the routines in Chapters 6, 7 and 8, or, using any cardio machine, do a simple version of intervals: Just work your tail off for a couple of minutes to jack up your heart rate, then ease off for two minutes. Repeat this sequence for 30 minutes. Even while

The 101 Burn-Zone Diet

Meal Plan A: Restricted Calories & Carbs
Follow this plan for four days, then use Meal Plan B for the fifth day. On workout days, replace two meals (such as Meals 2 and 3 or Meals 4 and 5) with a preworkout meal (20–40 grams of whey protein within 30 minutes of your workout) and a postworkout meal (40–60 grams of whey protein and 20 ounces of Gatorade within 30 minutes after your workout).

DAY 1

Meal 1
12 egg whites
1 bowl oatmeal
   (about ½ cup dry)

Meal 2
8–10 oz. turkey breast
1 cup green beans

Meal 3
8–10 oz. chicken breast
2 cups shredded cabbage
   mixed with fat-free mayo
   and Splenda

Meal 4
40–60 g whey protein
1 low-fat bran muffin or
   1 apple

Meal 5
12 oz. chicken breast
2 cups wax beans

Meal 6 (before bed)
40–60 g casein protein

DAY 2

Meal 1
12 egg whites
2 pieces rye toast with
   sugar-free jam

Meal 2
1⅓ cups fat-free
cottage cheese
   mixed with Splenda

Meal 3
8–10 oz. chicken breast with
   barbecue sauce
1–2 cups cauliflower with
   butter-flavored sprinkles

Meal 4
40–60 g whey protein
1 bowl cream of rice
   cereal mixed with
   Splenda

Meal 5
12 oz. fish
2 cups broccoli

Meal 6 (before bed)
40–60 g casein protein

DAY 3

Meal 1
8 egg whites
4 oz. lean steak
10 oz. (medium) potato,
   chopped and grilled

Meal 2
8–10 oz. ground turkey breast
1 cup green beans
¼ cup salsa

Meal 3
8–10 oz. chicken breast with
   soy sauce
2 cups chopped onions and
   green peppers

Meal 4
40–60 g whey protein
2 slices rye toast with low-sugar
   jam or 1 banana

Meal 5
12 oz. shrimp
2–3 cups spaghetti squash with
   grated Parmesan cheese

Meal 6 (before bed)
40–60 g casein protein

working at the easier pace, your heart rate should remain high and you'll burn a lot of calories.

If you do your cardio first thing in the morning, it's better to weight-train later in the day, after your body has had ample time to recover. This ensures that you get two metabolic boosts in one day, plus it doesn't interfere with your body's growth hormone production, a side effect that can occur when weights immediately follow cardio.

For most, 30 minutes of cardio will suffice, as long as it's done with high intensity. However, you can bump that up to 45 minutes if your body can handle it. To determine this, assess your energy level at the 25-minute mark. If you feel fatigued, stick to 30 minutes. If you don't feel fatigued, then you can push yourself to 45 minutes. Just don't overdo it — you're working on a calorie deficit and you don't want to crash and burn.

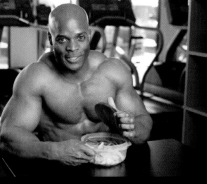

Meal Plan B: Higher Calories & Carbs

Use one of these options on Day 5, then start over on Meal Plan A for the next four days. If it's a training day, replace two meals (such as Meals 2 and 3 or Meals 4 and 5) with a preworkout meal (20–40 grams of whey protein and one piece of fruit within 30 minutes of your workout) and a postworkout meal (40–60 grams of whey protein and 20–32 ounces of Gatorade within 30 minutes after your workout).

DAY 4

Meal 1
8 egg whites
4 oz. ground turkey breast or
  low-fat turkey sausage
3 slices rye bread or
  1 bowl Cream of Rye
  cereal mixed
  with Splenda

Meal 2
50 g whey protein

Meal 3
8–10 oz. chicken breast with
  soy sauce
2 cups shredded cabbage mixed
  with fat-free mayo and Splenda

Meal 4
40–50 g whey protein
1 apple

Meal 5
12 oz. whitefish
2–3 cups mixed vegetables

Meal 6 (before bed)
40–60 g casein protein

DAY 5, Sample No. 1

Meal 1
8 egg whites
1 bowl oatmeal (about 1 cup dry)
1 banana

Meal 2
6 oz. turkey breast
1 cup brown rice

Meal 3
8 oz. chicken breast
1 cup carrots
1 small sweet potato

Meal 4
40–60 g whey protein
1 low-fat bran muffin or 1 apple

Meal 5
8 oz. chicken breast
1 kaiser roll
1 apple

Meal 6 (before bed)
40–60 g casein protein

DAY 5, Sample No. 2

Meal 1
8 egg whites
1 whole-wheat bagel with
  sugar-free jam

Meal 2
6 oz. chicken breast
1 cup cooked
  whole-wheat pasta
  with tomato sauce

Meal 3
8 oz. chicken breast
1 cup vegetables
1 small sweet potato

Meal 4
40–60 g whey protein
1 low-fat bran muffin or
  1 apple

Meal 5
8 oz. flank steak
1 medium baked potato with
  fat-free sour cream

Meal 6 (before bed)
40–60 g casein protein

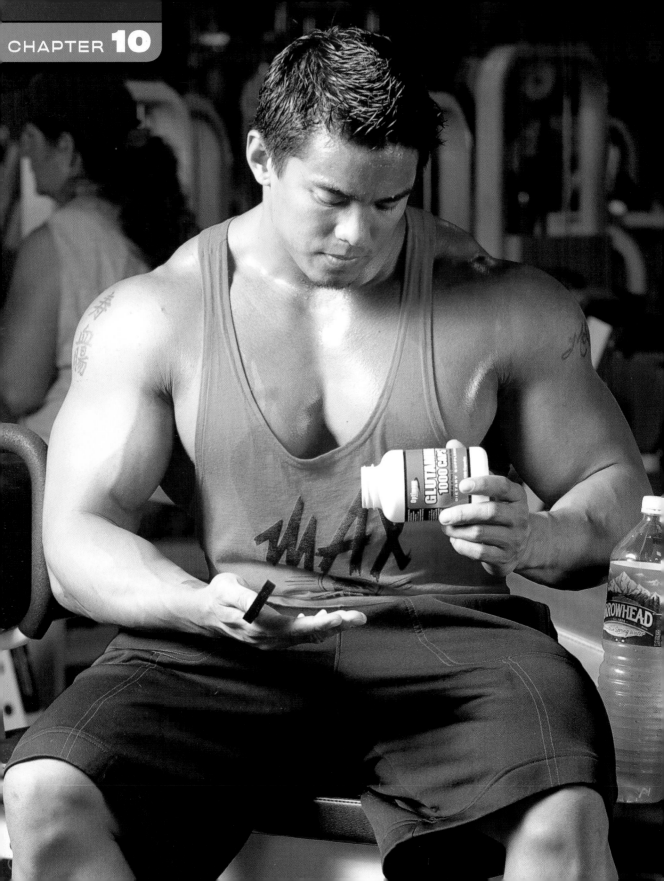

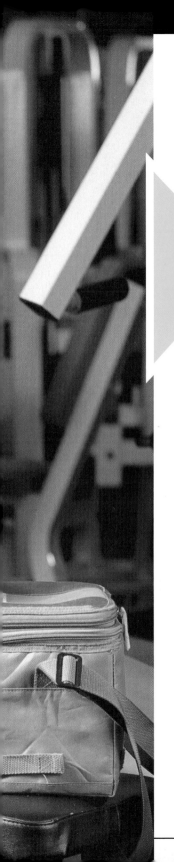

Around-The-Clock Gains

Scientific research shows that the best time of day to train may be in the early evening, when the body tends to be strongest and can burn the most calories and fat afterward. This is great news ... at least if you're a professional bodybuilder whose life revolves around working out. But what about the rest of us who are stuck lifting whenever we can cram it into our hectic schedules?

Although evening workouts may not be an option for you, you should, at least, be consistent about the time at which you train, whether that's first thing in the morning, on your lunch break or after a long day at the office. Being consistent is helpful, not only in terms of your training, but nutritionally, as well, because small dietary tweaks based on your specific workout time can make a world of difference in your results. Whether you train early, at midday or later on, this chapter has all of your nutritional conundrums covered.

EARLY BIRD FEELS THE BURN

If you train first thing in the morning, we've got two pieces of advice. First, don't work out on an empty stomach — we don't want you keeling over into a rack of dumbbells. Second, don't head to the gym after a big breakfast either, unless you fancy a second peek at your scrambled eggs mid-set. So what should you do? Shake up your morning. Be liquid. Powdered protein instead of the whole-food variety is the way to go. Here's how to map out your day.

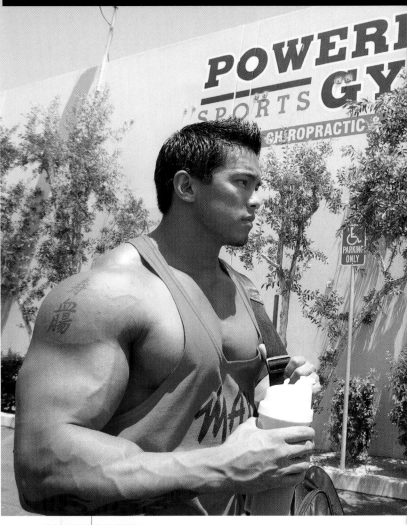

SUPPS FOR MORNING TRAINING

Timing your supplements and meals around a morning session can get a bit tricky. This plan takes the guesswork out of the "when" and "what," so you can get the most out of your early workouts.

1) When you wake

Place a bottle of arginine or other nitric oxide (NO) booster and a glass of water on your nightstand before bed. Take 3–5 grams of arginine as soon as you wake. This boosts NO levels and, therefore, blood flow and nutrients to the muscles during training. Then get ready for the gym.

FACT

10

>> grams of both whey and soy should be consumed before morning workouts

2) Preworkout

Guzzle down a 20-gram protein shake (10 grams of whey plus 10 grams of soy) along with 5–10 grams of branched-chain amino acids (BCAAs), 200–400 milligrams (mg) of caffeine and 3–5 grams of creatine, as well as 20–40 grams of slow-digesting carbs (oatmeal, whole-wheat toast, fruit, etc.) just before leaving the house. This stops the nighttime assault on your muscle mass, as the body breaks down muscle protein for fuel while you sleep.

Research shows that since testosterone levels are high when you wake, a protein shake and carb meal boosts the uptake of testosterone by the muscles and

Daily Meals for AM Workouts

How do you walk the line between eating too much and eating too little when you train in the morning? Follow this meal plan (and look to the text for supplements to take daily) for more productive workouts and faster results.

This sample diet plan is for a 160- to 200-pound morning trainee looking to gain lean mass and keep bodyfat off. If you're above or below this weight range, adjust the values accordingly. Shoot for about 8 calories, 1.5 grams of protein, 2 grams of carbs and 0.5 gram of fat per pound of bodyweight per day.

MEAL 1: Preworkout	MEAL 6: Snack
10 g whey protein + 10 g soy protein 1 large orange	1 cup low-fat cottage cheese ½ cup sliced pineapple 6 whole-wheat crackers
MEAL 2: Postworkout	**MEAL 7: Dinner**
40 g whey protein 32 oz. Gatorade	9 oz. broiled or grilled salmon 1 cup cooked brown rice
MEAL 3: Breakfast	2 cups broccoli
2 whole eggs 4 egg whites 2 cups cooked oatmeal	2 cups mixed green salad 2 Tbsp. olive oil/vinegar dressing
MEAL 4: Snack	**MEAL 8:** **Nighttime Snack**
20 g whey protein 1 medium banana 1 Tbsp. peanut butter	20 g casein protein 1 oz. mixed nuts
MEAL 5: Lunch	
1 can white tuna 1 Tbsp. fat-free mayonnaise 2 slices whole-wheat bread 1 cup blueberries	**TOTALS:** 3,392 calories, 299 g protein, 333 g carbs, 96 g fat **NOTE:** Mix all protein shakes in water per directions

increases the number of testosterone receptors in muscle cells. This means more test can do its job of boosting muscle mass.

Protein and carbs provide you with energy for your workout, and the soy in your protein shake further boosts NO and blood flow. Ax the carbs completely if you're trying to get lean and will do cardio after you hit the weights — the protein alone is sufficient for your fat-fighting effort.

Taking caffeine right before you train can significantly boost muscle strength and your ability to push your workouts to the limit. Take the aforementioned 200–400-mg dose as a caffeine supplement or 2–3 cups of brewed black coffee.

3) Immediately postworkout

Right after the last rep of your last set, take another 3–5-gram dose of arginine to boost recovery and push muscle growth. Then hit the showers and get ready for the workday ahead.

4) On your way to work

Now it's time to start the rebuilding process. Approximately 30 minutes after your postworkout arginine dose, drink a 40-gram whey shake along with 5–10 grams of BCAAs, 3–5 grams of creatine and 40–80 grams of fast-digesting carbs (Gatorade is a great choice). This flood of critical supplements kick-starts the muscle-growth process known as protein synthesis. Try to get this done before you get behind the wheel.

5) At your desk

Roughly 45–60 minutes after your postworkout shake, it's finally time for your actual breakfast. Go with 30–40 grams of a lean protein source such as six egg whites with a couple of yolks, chicken breast, lean beef or low-fat cottage cheese, and about 40 grams of slow-digesting carbs from sources such as oatmeal, whole-wheat bread, fruit or a sweet potato.

THE MIDDAY MUSCLE PLAN

If you train at lunchtime, it helps to have a job that allows you to eat your meals when you're not on your lunch break. Similar to the morning lifter, you want to bookend your gym session with protein shakes and grab a whole-food meal about an hour after your postworkout shake. That means you'll need to be prepared to eat at your workstation.

SUPPS FOR NOON TRAINING

Since you're better off taking some supps with food and others on an empty stomach, figuring out which ones to take and when can get pretty tricky if you're a noontime trainee. This plan helps you work with your eating and training schedule so your supps can get to the task of making you bigger and leaner.

1) When you wake

Consume a 20-gram protein shake (10 grams of whey plus 10 grams of soy), 5–10 grams of BCAAs and some fruit, which provides 20–30 grams of carbs. This stops the overnight breakdown of muscle mass and puts more of your testosterone to work boosting muscle growth. The soy also increases NO levels and blood flow so more of the amino acids from the whey can get to your muscles. After that, go take your shower — the first step is finished.

2) Before work

Have a big breakfast 30–60 minutes after your shake and fruit. Go with 30–40 grams of a quality protein source such as six egg whites with 2–3 yolks and 40–60 grams of slow-digesting carbs (oatmeal or whole-wheat toast work well). The slow-digesting carbs provide long-lasting energy and allow you to maximize

Meals for Noon Workouts

Follow this meal plan to make lunchtime a power hour for you every day. (See the text for supps.)

This sample diet plan is for a 160- to 200-pound lunchtime trainee looking to gain lean mass and keep bodyfat off. If you're above or below this weight range, adjust the values accordingly. Shoot for about 18 calories, 1.5 grams of protein, 2 grams of carbs and 0.5 gram of fat per pound of bodyweight per day.

MEAL 1: Early meal	MEAL 6: Snack
10 g whey protein + 10 g soy protein	1 cup low-fat cottage cheese
1 cup blueberries	½ cup sliced pineapple
MEAL 2: Breakfast	6 whole-wheat crackers
3 whole eggs	**MEAL 7: Dinner**
3 egg whites	9 oz. broiled or grilled salmon
2 cups cooked oatmeal	1 cup cooked brown rice
MEAL 3: Preworkout	2 cups broccoli
10 g whey protein + 10 g soy protein	2 cups mixed green salad
1 large orange	2 Tbsp. olive oil/vinegar dressing
MEAL 4: Postworkout	**MEAL 8: Nighttime Snack**
40 g whey protein	20 g casein protein
32 oz. Gatorade	1 oz. mixed nuts
MEAL 5: Lunch	
1 can white tuna	**TOTALS:** 3,333 calories, 297 g protein, 324 g carbs, 93 g fat
1 Tbsp. fat-free mayonnaise	
2 slices whole-wheat bread	**NOTE:** Mix all protein shakes in water per directions on label.
1 cup blueberries	

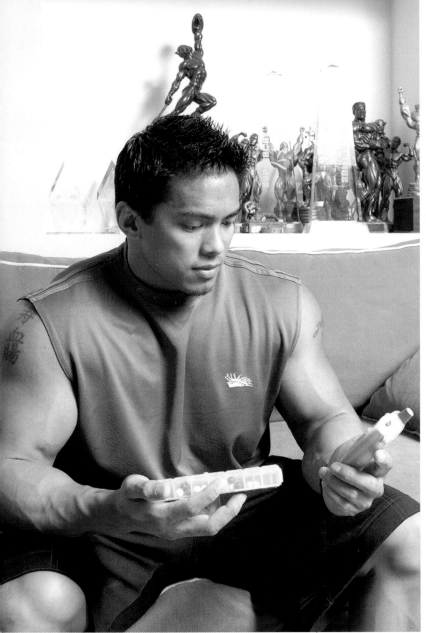

4) 30 minutes preworkout

Guzzle down a 20-gram mixed protein shake (10 grams of whey plus 10 grams of soy) with 5–10 grams of BCAAs, 3–5 grams of creatine and 20–40 grams of slow-digesting carbs. This combo gives you energy during the workout, and the soy further boosts NO and blood flow. (If you're trying to get lean and will do cardio after weights, either reduce or omit the carbs.)

Caffeine gives you a pick-me-up before you head to the gym by increasing muscle strength, so take in 200–400 mg in supplement form or drink 2–3 cups of black coffee.

5) Immediately postworkout

Once you knock out your final rep, take another 3–5-gram dose of arginine to boost recovery and drive muscle growth.

6) 30 minutes postworkout

This is when the real growth starts. About 30 minutes after your arginine dose, have a 40-gram whey protein shake, 5–10 grams of BCAAs, 3–5 grams of creatine and 40–80 grams of fast-digesting carbs.

fat-burning throughout the day to stay lean while packing on muscle.

3) One hour preworkout

Take 3–5 grams of arginine. This will boost NO levels and therefore blood flow and nutrient delivery to your muscles during the workout.

7) 45–60 minutes postworkout

Hungry? You should be. Eat a lunch consisting of 30–40 grams of a lean protein source and about 40 grams of slow-digesting carbs.

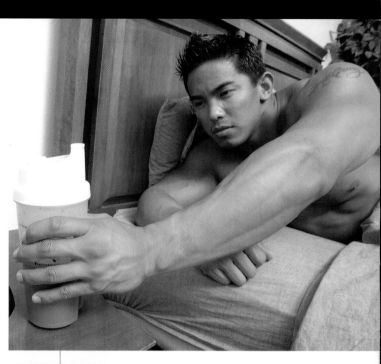

EVENING-TIME LIFTERS

If the crowded gyms are any indication, this is a very popular time to train. Unfortunately, one problem with training late in the day is getting a healthy portion of fast-digesting carbs postworkout. But cutting back on carbs at night is essential to reducing bodyfat, so this puts you in a tough spot.

The best solution, though, is actually pretty easy — don't go overboard with your carbohydrate consumption. Some carbs are necessary to keep your muscle growth on track; about 30–40 grams postworkout should do the trick.

In addition, while some type of stimulant or thermogenic is almost universally recommended preworkout, be wary of taking one if you train in the evening — there's nothing more miserable than a sleepless night when you have an early morning the next day. Look out for other supps that may have stimulants.

SUPPS FOR NIGHT TRAINING

As with the other trainees outlined earlier in this chapter, your supplement and meal timing should be dictated by the time of day you get to the gym. When you work out in the evening, there's less concentration on supplements early in the day, save for the requisite protein shakes.

FACT

3

>> minimum number of grams of arginine you should take before and after workouts

1) When you wake

It's a familiar refrain. As soon as your alarm goes off, take in a 20-gram whey/soy mixed protein shake, 5–10 grams of BCAAs and a piece of fruit providing 20–30 grams of carbs. Again, this halts the muscle-eating mode your body has slipped into overnight and maximizes the use of testosterone in your bloodstream. The soy increases NO levels, thereby getting the aminos and protein to your muscles more efficiently.

2) Before work

Have a big breakfast 30–60 minutes after your shake and fruit. Aim for at least 30–40 grams of protein — think six egg whites with 2–3 yolks — and 40–60 grams of slow-digesting carbs. This combination provides your brain and body with energy for the morning and keeps you feeling full longer.

3) One hour preworkout

Take 3–5 grams of arginine from an NO booster to enhance blood flow to the muscles during training. Depending on how late you work out and how soon afterward you go to bed, you may want to make sure your NO booster doesn't contain caffeine.

Meals for Late-Night Workouts

When you train late in the day, everything you eat leading up to your workout goes straight into the fuel tank. That's why, to stay anabolic 24/7, it's important to eat (and supplement) well around the time you train and throughout the day.

This sample diet plan is for a 160- to 200-pound evening trainee looking to gain lean mass and keep bodyfat off. If you're above or below this weight range, adjust accordingly. Shoot for about 18 calories, 1.5 grams of protein, 2 grams of carbs and 0.5 gram of fat per pound of bodyweight per day.

MEAL 1: Early meal	MEAL 6: Dinner
10 g whey protein + 10 g soy protein	9 oz. broiled or grilled salmon
1 cup blueberries	1 cup cooked brown rice
MEAL 2: Breakfast	2 cups broccoli
3 whole eggs	2 cups mixed green salad
3 egg whites	2 Tbsp. olive oil/ vinegar dressing
2 cups cooked oatmeal	**MEAL 7: Preworkout**
MEAL 3: Snack	10 g whey protein + 10 g soy protein
1 scoop whey protein	1 large orange
1 medium banana	**MEAL 8: Postworkout**
1 Tbsp. peanut butter	40 g whey protein
MEAL 4: Lunch	20 oz. Gatorade
1 can white tuna	**MEAL 9: Nighttime Snack**
1 Tbsp. fat-free mayonnaise	1 scoop casein protein
2 slices whole-wheat bread	
1 cup blueberries	**TOTALS:** 3,304 calories, 317 g protein, 317 g carbs, 86 g fat
MEAL 5: Snack	**NOTE:** Mix all protein shakes in water per directions on label.
1 cup low-fat cottage cheese	
½ cup sliced pineapple	
6 whole-wheat crackers	

4) 30 minutes preworkout

About a half-hour before your workout, guzzle down a 20-gram protein shake, again made with 10 grams of whey and 10 grams of soy. Also, take 5–10 grams of BCAAs and 3–5 grams of creatine, along with 20–40 grams of slow-digesting carbs. The carbs are especially crucial for energy levels if you're forgoing a stimulant-boosted NO product.

A 200- to 400-mg dose of caffeine is usually recommended in this window, but since you're a nighttime trainee you have to be honest with yourself: How do you tolerate it? Research shows that caffeine taken right before training can significantly boost muscle strength and it can also positively affect your ability to push your workouts to the limit, but it might not be worth it if you end up staring at the ceiling all night. If you're sensitive to caffeine and it interferes with sleep, nix it.

5) Immediately postworkout

Time for more arginine — definitely of the nonstimulant variety, per the above notes on tolerance. Go for 3–5 grams of NO here.

6) 30 minutes postworkout

Put down a 40-gram whey protein shake now; taking your whey any sooner will counteract the benefits of your arginine. Also, get in 5–10 grams of BCAAs, 3–5 grams of creatine and — say it with us — 30–40 grams of fast-digesting carbs from a source such as Gatorade. If this meal comes within two hours of sleep, replace 20 grams of whey with 20 grams of casein protein containing micellar casein and skip the next step.

7) 45–60 minutes postworkout

Drink a 20-gram casein shake containing micellar casein. This slow-digesting protein supplies a slow and steady trickle of amino acids throughout the night, preventing the body from breaking down muscle protein for fuel.

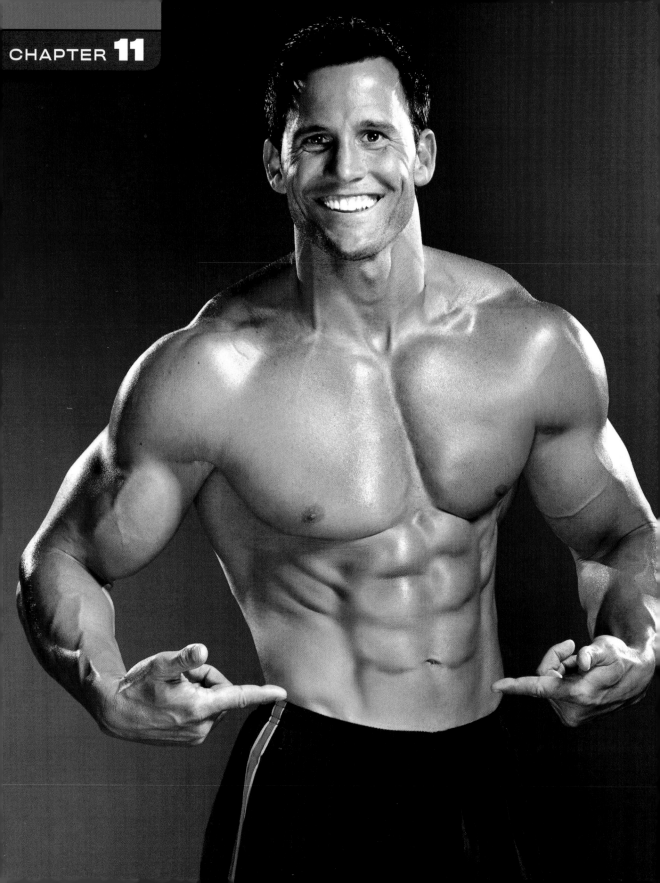

Top Nine Combos For Fat Loss

You've heard the old phrase two heads are better than one? The same logic applies to many things: socks, hundred-dollar bills and Beyoncé Knowles, to name but a few.

The edict also holds true for supplements in many cases. Where one supplement can help your body burn fat, using it along with one or more others can really ramp up the overall effects. Taking full advantage of this synergy not only gets you more bang for your supplement buck, but also helps you reach your physique goals faster.

With that exciting prospect in mind, check out the following nine supplement combinations outlined in this chapter. They may provide that extra fat-burning edge you're looking for.

THE CHEAPSKATE COMBO: CAFFEINE AND GREEN TEA EXTRACT

1 There are a lot of effective fat-burners on the market today, but for some people, such as college students and others on a tight budget, the sticker price alone can be more than they normally spend on food. But fat-loss supplements don't have to be expensive to be effective. Caffeine and green tea extract are in almost every fat-burner on the market today because they work well. If you purchase them alone without the bells and whistles, however, you'll find a potent fat-burner combo that costs you only pennies a day.

One of the major ways caffeine boosts fat loss is through its ability to bind to fat cells and enhance the removal of fat from them while inhibiting the storage of more fat. Caffeine also works to increase fat-burning during rest and exercise.

Green tea extract contains compounds known as catechins. One of them,

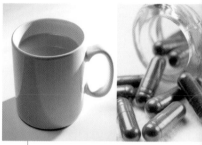

called epigallocate-chin gallate (EGCG), is responsible for the majority of green tea's fat-burning effects. EGCG has the ability to inhibit an enzyme that breaks down norepinephrine, the neurotransmitter involved in regulating metabolic rate and fat-burning. By stopping the breakdown of norepinephrine, you can keep metabolism and fat-burning elevated longer, especially when caffeine is used in conjunction with it. Research studies confirm that green tea extract can significantly boost fat loss.

Combine them like this: *In the morning and an hour before workouts, go with 200–400 mg of caffeine anhydrous (5–10 cents) with 500–1,000 mg of green tea extract standardized for EGCG (15–30 cents). On rest days, take a second dose in the afternoon. Total daily cost is about 40–80 cents.*

ONE-TWO FAT-FIGHTING PUNCH: FORSKOLIN AND CARNITINE

2 To maximize fat-burning, you need a supplement that goes directly to where fat is stored and frees it so it can travel in the bloodstream to muscles and other tissues of the body where it will be used for fuel. You also need to make sure the fat is carried into the machinery that burns it, the cell mitochondria. This supplement combo helps on both fronts.

Forskolin, the active compound in the herb *Coleus forskohlii*, gets the first half of the job done well, working to enhance fat loss by activating the enzyme adenylate cyclase. This enzyme causes a cascade of events that leads to the activation of another enzyme, hormone-sensitive lipase (HSL). HSL increases lipolysis, or the ability of the fat stored in fat cells to be released into the bloodstream, where it can travel to tissues such as muscle. In fact, one study from the University of Kansas (Lawrence) reported that overweight men who took forskolin lost significantly more bodyfat than test subjects who took a placebo during a 12-week study.

> **Overweight men who took forskolin lost more fat than a placebo group.**

Carnitine, an amino-acidlike supplement, helps the fat that gets to tissues travel into the mitochondria of those cells, where it's burned for fuel. Research confirms that carnitine supplementation improves fat-burning during exercise and rest, and leads to greater fat loss.

Combine them like this: *Take 20–50 mg of forskolin and 1–3 grams of carnitine (as L-carnitine, acetyl-L-carnitine or L-carnitine-L-tartrate) with breakfast, preworkout meals and postworkout meals.*

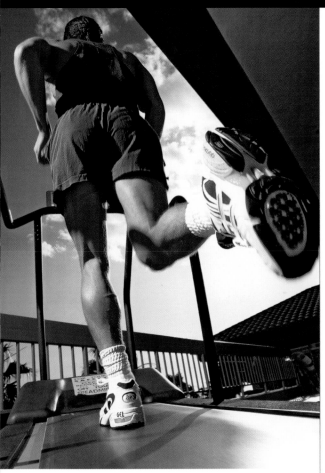

metabolic rate and lactic acid production by muscle. Since lactic acid stimulates growth hormone (GH) release and GH increases lipolysis, this is another fat-loss benefit of ginger.

Combine them like this: *Look for ways to add red pepper or ginger to your meals. Red pepper obviously goes well with traditional Mexican-style foods, but it can also be used to spice up eggs or cottage cheese. You could also use red pepper–based hot sauces and salsas on foods. An easy way to get ginger on your plate is next to your sushi or sashimi in the form of pickled ginger. You can also buy ginger root and slice it into a stir-fry, or use a generous portion of dried ginger.*

SPICE UP YOUR PHYSIQUE:
RED PEPPER AND GINGER

3 Sometimes increasing your body's fat-burning potential is as easy as using certain spices in your food. Adding a little red pepper or ginger is an easy way to spice up your meals and increase your metabolism.

If you like spicy food, then boosting fat loss can be as simple as eating. Capsaicin is the chemical in chili (red) peppers that makes them spicy. It boosts bodyfat loss by increasing metabolic rate and fat-burning through its ability to raise levels of norepinephrine. It also works to significantly decrease hunger and thus your overall caloric intake.

Ginger is a root with numerous properties that make it an effective treatment for inflammation, nausea and motion sickness. It's also a valuable aid for fat loss. Research shows that both fresh and dry ginger increase

GENETIC ENGINEERING: SESAMIN AND TTA

4 Some supplements work to enhance fat loss by increasing the activity of the genes that control fat-burning and fat storage. Sesamin and TTA are two such products.

Sesamin, a lignan from sesame oil, is a powerful antioxidant that's also a potent fat-burner. The active form of sesamin has been found to turn on a specific receptor (found in muscle, heart and liver cells) known as peroxisome proliferator-activated receptor alpha (PPAR alpha). Activating PPAR alpha turns on genes that increase fat-burning and

decrease fat storage.

Tetradecylthioacetic acid (TTA) is a specialized fatty acid that has sulfur bound to it, which prevents it from being burned for fuel by the body but allows it to regulate the burning and storage of dietary fats. TTA works by stimulating PPAR alpha as well as PPAR delta and PPAR gamma, providing other effects such as diminishing total cholesterol and LDL (bad) cholesterol levels while boosting insulin sensitivity. This means your body needs less insulin released than normal, which can further aid fat-loss efforts.

Combine them like this: *Take 500–1,000 mg of sesamin and 250–1,000 mg of TTA with breakfast, lunch and dinner.*

MINERAL MASH-UPS: CALCIUM, SELENIUM AND ZINC

5 Most guys think of minerals only as something with health benefits found in their multivitamin supplement. Yet several minerals are critical in your quest to become and stay lean. Getting ample amounts of these three will do the trick.

By now you may be familiar with the fact that calcium can help with fat loss and prevent fat gain. Calcium regulates the hormone calcitriol, which causes the body to produce fat and inhibits fat breakdown. When calcium levels are adequate, calcitriol is suppressed. Calcium also aids fat loss by decreasing the amount of dietary fat that's absorbed by your intestines.

The trace mineral selenium is critical for thyroid hormone production, and is a component of the enzyme that helps convert the thyroid hormone thyroxine (T4) to triiodothyronine (T3), which keeps metabolism elevated. Low selenium levels can impair thyroid function and promote hypo-thyroidism, or low levels of thyroid hormones.

Zinc is important because being low in this mineral can interfere with thyroid hormone production, leading to a lowered metabolic rate, which makes it harder to drop bodyfat. Zinc deficiency is common in hard-training athletes, especially when they cut calories in an effort to get lean. One study from the University of Massachusetts (Amherst) found that subjects who were on a low-zinc diet had significantly slower metabolic rates. When they took a zinc supplement (25 mg) for 20 days, their metabolisms jumped to higher levels than before they followed a low-zinc diet. A recent study from Andong National University (South Korea) showed that zinc deficiency lowered levels of leptin, a hormone that keeps metabolism elevated and hunger suppressed.

Combine them like this: *Take about 1,000 mg of calcium and 200–400 micrograms (mcg) of selenium per day with food. The best way to take zinc is as ZMA on an empty stomach before bed; the 30 mg of zinc in it provides insurance against slow metabolism syndrome.*

BONUS COMBO: EGGS & OATMEAL

If you think eating certain foods can't enhance your fat-loss capabilities, you're in for a pleasant surprise. The more we learn about nutrition, the more functional foods — those that provide specific functions in our bodies — we discover. Some of these foods are perfect for stimulating fat loss, such as these two heavy hitters.

Eggs, and the nearly perfect protein they contain, not only help you pack on quality muscle mass but are proven to help with fat loss as well. One study found that having eggs for breakfast reduced hunger and food intake for more than 24 hours compared to a breakfast containing bagels. A 2007 longer-term follow-up study performed at Louisiana State University's Pennington Biomedical Research Center (Baton Rouge) revealed that those who consumed two eggs at breakfast at least five times per week for eight weeks lost significantly more weight and more fat around their waistlines than those who ate a bagel instead.

Oatmeal and other slow-digesting carbs (such as whole-wheat bread) will aid bodyfat loss by keeping insulin levels steady and increasing the amount of fat you burn during the day. Research from Loughborough University (UK) reported that when athletes ate slow-digesting carbs at breakfast and lunch, they had lower insulin levels and higher fat-burning during the day compared to those who ate fast-digesting carbs. They also found that those who ate slow carbohydrates burned more fat during exercise and were able to exercise longer.

>> **Combine them like this:** For breakfast, have three whole eggs and three egg whites along with 1 cup of cooked oatmeal or two slices of whole-wheat toast.

AMINO ACID BURN: GLUTAMINE AND ARGININE

6 Amino acids are the building blocks of protein, and a few provide potent anabolic effects. But did you know that some also have impressive fat-burning properties? Glutamine and arginine are two such amino acids, and their fat-burning effects are magnified when they're combined.

Research shows that glutamine can increase fat-burning and metabolic rate. In a study from Iowa State University (Ames), test subjects who took glutamine with breakfast increased the number of calories and amount of fat burned for energy compared to when they took an amino acid mixture (glycine, serine and alanine). In a follow-up study from the same lab,

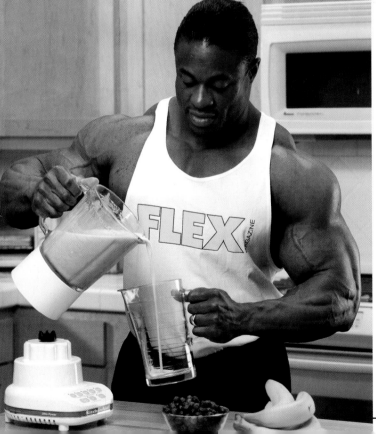

scientists showed that glutamine taken before exercise resulted in more calories being burned than when subjects took the aforementioned amino mixture. In addition, glutamine is effective at boosting GH. Although GH is very anabolic, it also works to increase lipolysis, which frees fat from fat cells.

Arginine's ability to boost nitric oxide levels is well known, but that same property also makes it a quality fat-burner. Research shows that NO can increase fat-burning due to its ability to enhance lipolysis. With the greater metabolic burn from glutamine, the freed fat is much more likely to be burned for fuel. Also, arginine increases GH release, which enhances lipolysis. Confirmation of the ability of arginine to improve fat loss came in a 2007 study from the University of North Carolina (Wilmington) that showed that female athletes who supplemented with arginine for four weeks lost bodyfat and simultaneously gained muscle mass without otherwise changing their dietary intakes.

Combine them like this: *Take 5–10 grams of glutamine with breakfast, before and after workouts and before bed. Take 3–10 grams of arginine (as L-arginine, arginine alpha-ketoglutarate, arginine ketoisocaproate, arginine mallate or arginine ethyl ester) 30–60 minutes before breakfast, 30–60 minutes before workouts, immediately after workouts and 30–60 minutes before bed.*

POTENT PROTEIN: WHEY AND SOY

7 You probably know the importance of using protein powders for stimulating muscle growth, but did you realize they can also encourage fat loss? Using whey and soy protein powders to supplement your protein needs is a great way to strip away bodyfat while maximizing muscle growth.

Several studies show that bodyfat loss is

enhanced when the diet is supplemented with whey protein powder. One major reason for this may be due to whey's ability to significantly decrease hunger. A study from the University of Surrey (UK) found that subjects who drank a whey protein shake 90 minutes before eating a buffet meal ate significantly less food than when they instead drank a casein protein shake. The reason for this appears to be the 60% greater rise in the hunger-blunting hormones cholecystokinin and glucagon-like peptide-1 that comes after whey is ingested.

If you're up on your protein information, you know that soy isn't just a protein for women — it has numerous benefits for male bodybuilders. One is enhanced fat loss. Research from the University of Illinois (Champaign-Urbana) has discovered that soy protein contains peptides (small proteins) that influence the brain to keep your resting metabolic rate elevated to help burn more bodyfat, as well as decrease hunger to help you eat fewer calories throughout the day.

Combine them like this: *Immediately before workouts, drink a shake containing 10 grams each of whey and soy proteins. Right after workouts, drink a shake containing 20 grams each of whey and soy protein powders. In between meals, snack on a shake containing 10–20 grams each of whey and soy proteins.*

HUNGER HELPER: GLUCOMANNAN AND 5-HTP

8 Face it: To get lean, you have to drop calories and carbs. But one problem with this solution is the hunger that comes with it. The good news is that some supplements can help keep hunger at bay.

Glucomannan, a soluble fiber derived from the root of the konjac plant, absorbs a large amount of water in the digestive tract, causing you to feel full. One study from the University of Connecticut (Storrs) found that subjects who supplemented with glucomannan lost significant amounts of weight and fat whether or not they exercised.

For some guys, dropping carbs is a difficult task. Serotonin levels tend to dip when dieting, especially with a lower carb intake. This prompts strong carb cravings, especially at night. The essential amino acid tryptophan gets converted into 5-hydroxytryptophan (5-HTP) before it forms serotonin and melatonin in the body, which will help curb your carb cravings and relax you before bed. One study from the University of Rome found that obese subjects who took 5-HTP ate fewer calories per day and lost 11 pounds in 12 weeks; test subjects who took a placebo reported that they had difficulty limiting their food intake and lost only 2 pounds.

Combine them like this: *Take 1–2 grams of glucomannan before meals and 50–300 mg of 5-HTP in the evenings.*

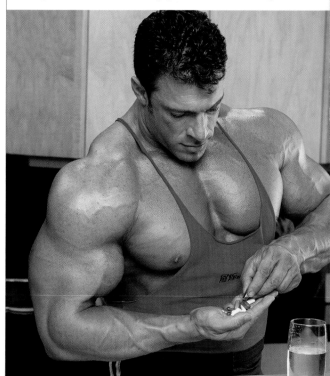

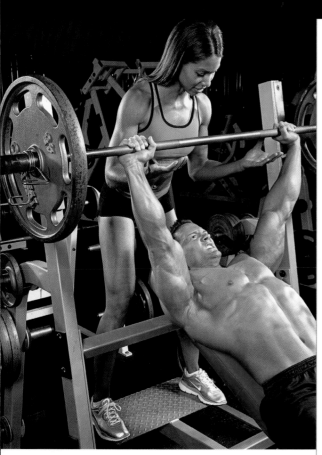

FATTY ACID BURN: CLA AND FISH OIL

9 Twenty years ago, when everyone was stressing the importance of a low-fat diet void of all kinds of fat, the term *healthy fat* was virtually unknown. Back then, doctors, scientists and nutritionists recommended staying away from nuts, avocados, olive oil, salmon and many of the other fat sources we now know we should include in our diets. Suggesting that taking fats can

help you drop fat may still seem paradoxical to some, yet the following two fat sources will do just that when taken as directed.

Conjugated linoleic acid (CLA) has been proven in numerous clinical trials to help shed bodyfat while adding muscle mass as well as boosting strength. One way that CLA works is by inhibiting lipoprotein lipase, an enzyme found around fat cells that seemingly is tasked to pick up fat from the circulation and store it as bodyfat. One study found that subjects who supplemented

with CLA for six months without dieting or exercising lost more bodyfat (with the majority coming from the waist) than those who took an equal amount of olive oil. The CLA group also managed to gain muscle mass without exercising. Another study, from the University of Saskatchewan (Saskatoon, Canada), reported that subjects who took CLA while following a weight-training program lost more bodyfat and gained more muscle mass and strength without dieting than subjects who took a placebo.

Fish oil contains the

essential omega-3 fatty acids, which are now known to be beneficial for burning fat. One of the main mechanisms is through the conversion of omega-3s to beneficial prostaglandins — hormonelike substances that can promote thermogenesis. A study from Virginia Commonwealth University (Richmond) found that omega-3 fatty acids also help prevent dietary fat from being stored as bodyfat.

Combine them like this: *Take 2–3 grams of CLA and 1–2 grams of fish oil with breakfast, lunch and dinner.*

> ## Conjugated linoleic acid has been proven in numerous trials to help shed bodyfat.

COMBINING THE COMBOS

Although choosing one effective fat-burning combination from our list will help you shed fat, you can combine the combos for additive results. Your best bet is to employ all nine combinations if you can afford it. We suggest you start with the simplest ones such as Combos 2, 4, 5 and 9. Try them for several weeks, then add other combos one at a time such as Combo 3, then 1, 6, 7 and 8 if needed. Along with training and diet, it should all add up to one great physique.

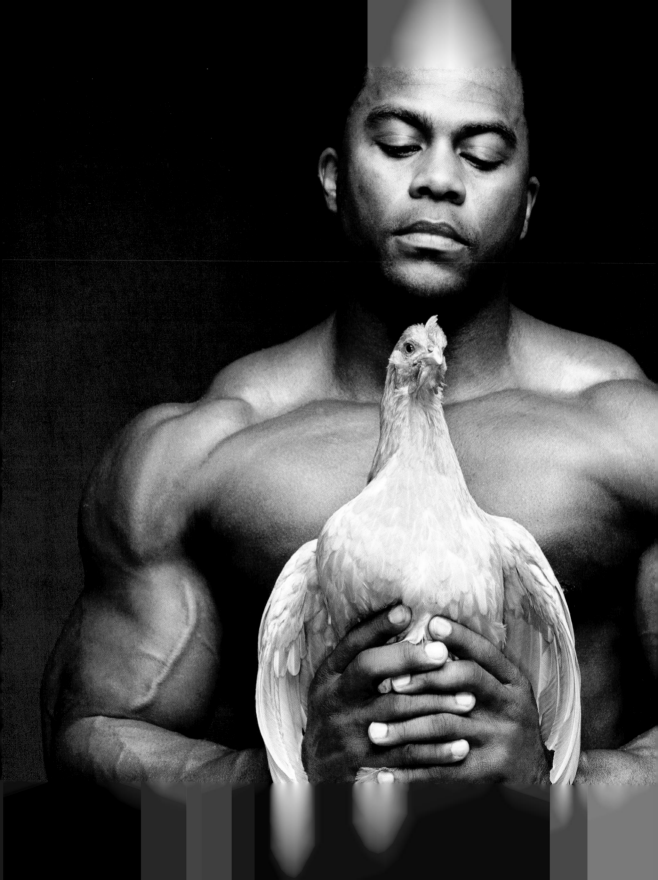

The Shell Game

Rocky Balboa downed pitchers of them

like a contestant on *Fear Factor*. Jay Cutler, the Mr. Olympia champion in 2006 and 2007, has been known to devour up to two dozen a day. And for many of us, they're the only thing that goes with an order of turkey sausage on a Sunday morning.

Of course, we're talking about eggs, an unflagging and essential staple of every bodybuilder's (and wannabe bodybuilder's) diet.

It almost goes without saying that eggs are nutritious. But do you know why they're so darn good for you? In the following pages, we give you all the facts you need to know, and tell you how to prepare eggs in the kitchen for optimal flavor too. Consider this your complete guide to one of nature's most perfect foods.

EGG HEAD |
Q&A

We've all wondered how flexible an egg's expiration date is. Expand your knowledge with answers to that and eight other common questions about eggs.

Q Which grade of eggs is the best?
Grade AA is best. However, there's little difference between A and AA.

Q Does size matter?
The size of an egg doesn't affect its taste, but it does affect its nutrients — a larger egg has more protein and calories.

Q What are the main differences between brown and white eggs?
The color of an eggshell is determined by the breed of hen that laid the egg. White hens lay white eggs, while their red-feathered relatives lay brown ones.

Q What does it mean when an egg yolk has a blood spot?
Blood spots on egg yolks are caused by a blood vessel rupturing on the yolk while the egg is being formed. These spots are rare — electronic sensors usually detect them — and perfectly safe to ingest.

Q Can you eat eggs after their "sell by" date?
If stored properly in the fridge, eggs should still taste fine and be safe to eat up to two weeks after their "sell by" date.

Q What is an organic vs. a free-range egg?
Organic eggs are produced by hens fed a diet free of pesticides, fungicides, herbicides and commercial fertilizers. Free-range eggs are produced by hens raised outdoors or that have daily access to the outdoors.

Q Are organic and free-range eggs more healthful than regular eggs?
All of these eggs have the same number of calories and macronutrients. However, some eggs are laid by hens fed a special diet that increases the micronutrients in their eggs. Eggs from Eggland's Best, for example, contain more omega-3 fatty acids, vitamin E and lutein than regular eggs.

Q Why does a hard-boiled yolk sometimes look green?
Yolks turn green when they're overcooked or when there's a lot of iron in the cooking water. It doesn't affect the nutrients or flavor.

Q What are Egg Beaters made of?
Pasteurized egg whites, added vitamins and minerals, and beta-carotene to give them a yellow hue.

FACT 67
>> percentage of an egg's liquid weight that is egg white

FIT FOOD

WHETHER YOU'RE TRYING TO ADD MASS OR GET LEAN, eggs are a nearly perfect food. A large one contains 75 calories, 4 grams of fat and 6 grams of protein. Lose the yolks and you've got just 17 calories and zero grams of fat, with 4 grams of protein. Eggs also contain more than 15 amino acids, including arginine and leucine, and omega-3 fatty acids.

Despite nutritional concerns that came to a head in the 1990s, it turns out that even cholesterol-watchers don't have to subsist on egg whites alone. Studies show that a healthy man can eat up to two yolks a day without impacting his blood cholesterol level. And since the yolk contains valuable nutrients such as vitamins A, D, E and B_{12} that aren't found in egg whites, they won't just make for a tastier omelet but a healthier one, as well.

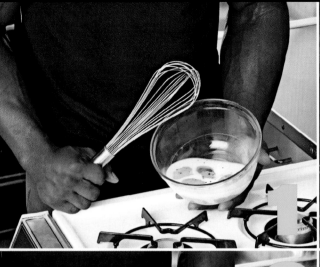
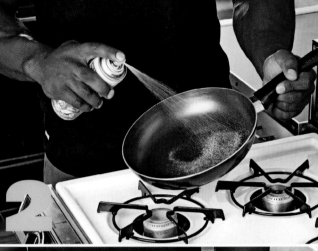
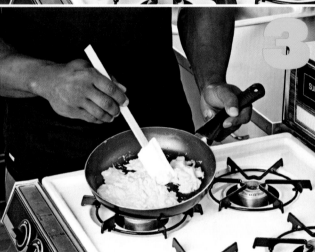
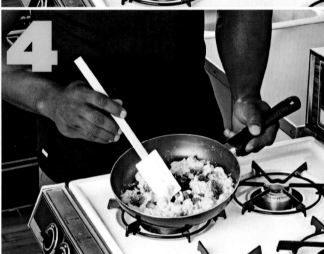

1 2
3 4

Get Cooking

HOW TO SCRAMBLE, ETC., WITHOUT GETTING EGG ON YOUR FACE

TECHNIQUE Scrambled Eggs

For a heartier scramble, toss in a handful of vegetables, low-fat cheese or chopped cooked chicken breast halfway through cooking.

You'll need: A bowl, 8- to 10-inch omelet pan or skillet, whisk, rubber spatula, 4 eggs, 4 tablespoons fat-free milk, ⅛ teaspoon salt, dash of pepper, nonstick cooking spray

STEP 1 In a bowl, beat together eggs, milk, salt and pepper with a whisk.

STEP 2 Spray a pan heated over medium heat with nonstick cooking spray. Put a drop of water in the pan to check the temperature — the water should sizzle. Pour egg mixture into the pan.

STEP 3 As the eggs begin to set, use a spatula to scrape the sides of the pan, forming large clumps.

STEP 4 Continue cooking until no visible liquid remains.

>> TIP Egg whites take longer to cook than whole eggs because they contain more water.

>> TIP To save yourself the labor of cracking and separating eggs for egg whites, try a pasteurized egg product such as All Whites.

1

2

3

4

TECHNIQUE Omelet

An omelet makes an easy dinner: Just add a side salad or baked sweet potato.

You'll need: A bowl, 4 eggs, 4 tablespoons fat-free milk or water, 8- to 10-inch omelet pan or skillet, whisk, flexible spatula or pancake turner, ⅛ teaspoon salt, dash of pepper, nonstick cooking spray

STEP 1 In a bowl, beat together eggs, milk or water, salt and pepper with a whisk.

STEP 2 Heat a pan over medium-high heat, spray with nonstick cooking spray and add a drop of water — it should sizzle when it hits the pan. Pour in the egg mixture.

STEP 3 With a spatula, push the edges of the mixture toward the center so the uncooked egg reaches the pan. (You may need to tilt the pan as well.)

STEP 4 When no visible liquid remains, top half of the mixture with desired filling ingredients. Fold the unfilled portion over the filled portion, and carefully slide omelet onto a plate.

>> TIP If you're using just whites, use six but keep the amount of milk or water the same.

>> TIP You can fill an omelet with almost any food. Be sure you heat refrigerator-cold foods to serving temperature or fully cook raw foods before cooking the omelet.

WHITES YOUR WAY

>> START WITH 4 egg whites + 2 tablespoons fat-free milk. Add one item from each column, plus salt and pepper to taste

1 TSP.	¼ CUP	⅛ CUP
basil	sliced mushrooms	shredded cheddar cheese
thyme	chopped tomatoes	
chives	chopped spinach (fresh or frozen)	grated parmesan cheese
cilantro	broccoli	part-skim mozzarella cheese
tarragon	diced onions and peppers (equal parts)	Jack cheese

Top it off with one of these: ¼ cup prepared salsa; ¼ cup cottage cheese; half a medium avocado, sliced

>> Flexible spatula A silicone spatula will have you flipping omelets like a pro.

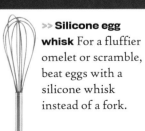

>> Silicone egg whisk For a fluffier omelet or scramble, beat eggs with a silicone whisk instead of a fork.

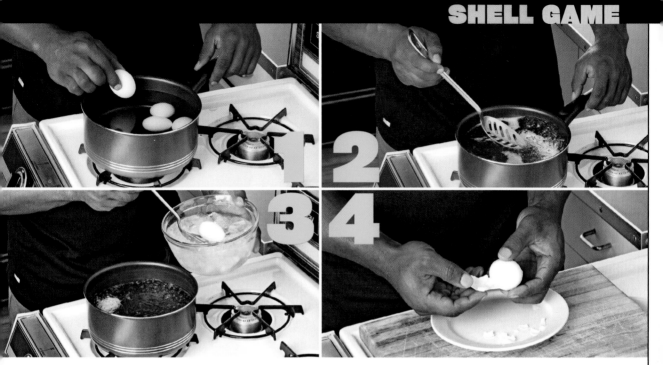

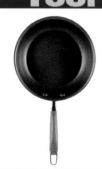

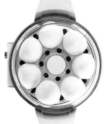

TECHNIQUE
Hard-Boiling

The best way to hard-boil an egg is by not overboiling it! You'll eliminate cracked eggs and overcooking by starting with cold water.

You'll need: A large saucepan, eggs, water, spoon

STEP 1 Place eggs in a saucepan large enough to allow them to cook in a single layer. Add enough cold water to cover the eggs by 1–2 inches.

STEP 2 Heat the pot, uncovered, over high heat until the water comes to a rolling boil. Then reduce the heat to low and cook eggs an additional 10 minutes. Water should continue to boil gently.

STEP 3 Remove the pot from heat and run eggs under cold water or spoon them into a bowl of ice water until completely cooled.

STEP 4 Either peel and eat eggs immediately or store in the refrigerator for up to one week.

>> **TIP** Add a few drops of food coloring to the water when you hard-boil eggs. The shells will end up slightly colored, making them easy to distinguish from raw eggs in your fridge.

Egg yolks are one of the few foods that naturally contain vitamin D.

Tool School | STOCK YOUR KITCHEN WITH THESE GADGETS AND MAKE A PERFECT EGG EVERY TIME

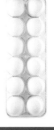

>> **Nonstick frying pan** The nonstick surface means you'll need just a spritz of cooking spray to make the perfect omelet.

>> **Egg cooker** Too lazy to time a pot of boiling water? A gadget like this can perfectly boil several eggs at once.

>> **Egg container** An airtight container keeps eggs fresher longer than cardboard cartons.

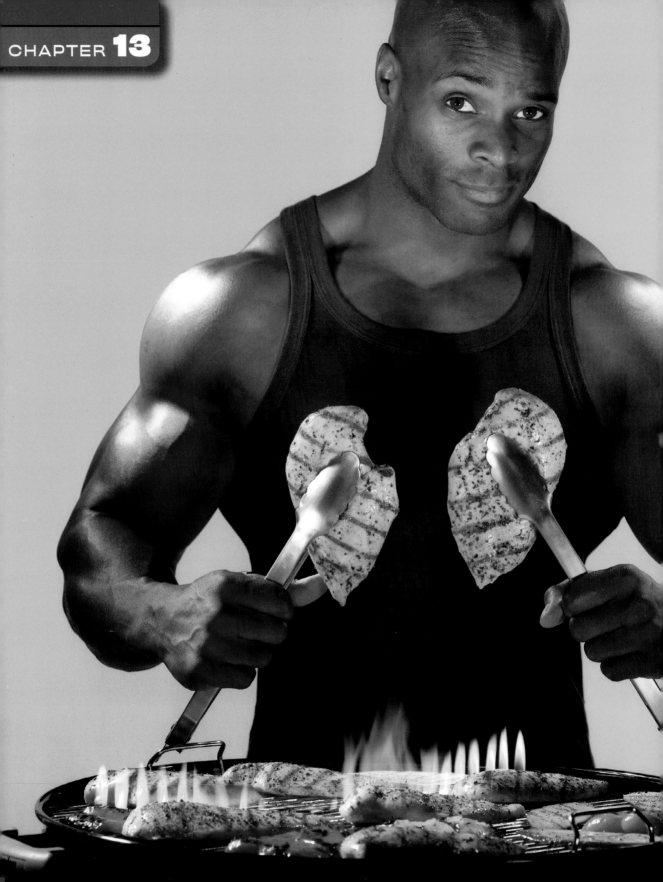

Your Protein Power Source

By design, working to make your muscle bigger and stronger is hard work. To successfully navigate the cycle of stress/recovery/growth, your muscles need all the help they can get. One way to accelerate that cycle is to eat the right amount of the right food at the right time.

Enter the chicken breast. Loaded with protein and other less-celebrated nutritional gems, this white-meat wonder is convenient, versatile and low in fat — no surprise, then, that it's the most common muscle-building food found on the dinner plates of gym rats everywhere. Yet day after day of the same old grilled chicken breast can make even the most die-hard bird-lover want to fly the coop.

To honor this classic bodybuilding food, we give you the skinny on why chicken breast deserves to be front-and-center in a healthful diet, and offer tasty secrets to bust you out of a chicken rut.

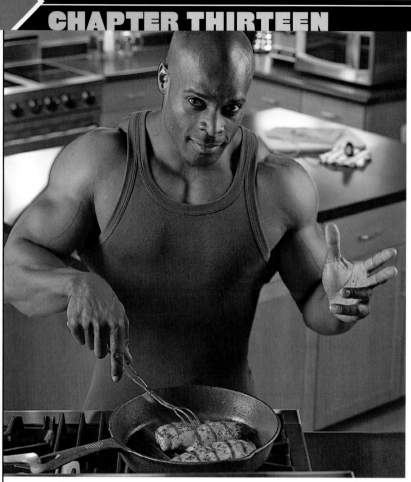

Vitamin B$_6$ allows you to use carbs (glycogen) stored in your muscles during exercise.

Iron is needed to deliver oxygen to those same muscles when you're training in overdrive.

Selenium repairs damaged cells and inhibits the growth of cancerous ones, helping to lower your risk of cancer. It also aids in proper thyroid function, which in turn helps keep your metabolism revving — another good reason to use chicken breast as a primary protein source when dieting.

Zinc is an immune-boosting mineral that can ward off cold bugs and support the production of anabolic hormones.

Just make sure that you enjoy your breast sans skin. If you eat it with the skin on, you get more than seven times the total fat and saturated fat content. It's okay to grill chicken with the skin on for flavor, but take it off before eating.

MUSCLE FOOD

With a higher protein-to-fat ratio (19:1) than any other part of the chicken, the breast is a great source of lean protein. And its protein quality ranks right up there with other heavyweights like eggs and beef, meaning it's easily synthesized to repair muscle tissue and other cells damaged during hard training. But there's more than just protein under those feathers: A 6-ounce chicken breast provides about 187 calories, 40 grams of protein, zero carbs and only 2 grams of fat along with a host of other bodybuilding-friendly nutrients.

Niacin is essential for the conversion of protein, fat and carbs into energy, and one chicken breast contains more than the recommended daily allowance of niacin. In other words, it can help you push more weight around in the gym and stay on the treadmill longer.

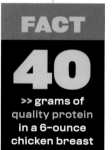

FACT

40

>> grams of quality protein in a 6-ounce chicken breast

A BETTER BIRD

Follow our six rules for buying, cooking and storing chicken breasts and you'll no longer have to needlessly suffer through tasteless, dried-out poultry.

RULE #1: Buy Organic

"I'm convinced that free-roaming, organic chicken is a better choice for bodybuilders [and other consumers] than those cooped up in factory farms. Plus, it's superior in taste," says chef Terrance Brennan, owner of Picholine restaurant in New York and author of *Artisanal Cooking* (Wiley & Sons, 2005).

Most other chefs agree, meaning the free-range birds are worth the extra expense. Brennan points out that industrialized chicken is often pumped full of water,

FOWL PLAY

FOR MARINADES, PICK ONE THAT'S TO YOUR TASTE AND REFRIGERATE EIGHT HOURS OR OVERNIGHT

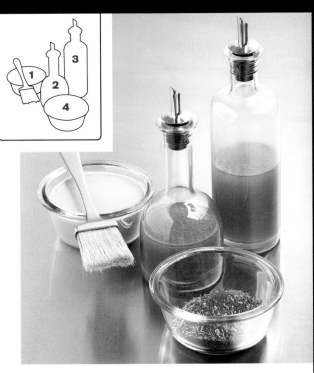

1) Tandoori Marinade

>> ¾ cup plain fat-free yogurt
>> ¾ Tbsp. ground coriander
>> ¾ Tbsp. paprika
>> ½ Tbsp. ground cumin
>> ½ Tbsp. ground ginger
>> 1 tsp. garlic powder
>> 1 tsp. ground black pepper
>> ½ tsp. ground cinnamon
>> ½ tsp. ground cardamom
>> ¼ tsp. ground cloves
>> Juice of ½ lemon

Mix all ingredients in a bowl. Pour over chicken and turn to coat. Set aside extra marinade to top cooked chicken.

NUTRITION FACTS
(¼-cup serving):
41 calories, 2 g protein, 8 g carbs, 1 g fat

2) Red Wine Marinade

>> ½ cup dry red wine
>> ¼ cup red wine vinegar
>> 2 garlic cloves, minced
>> 1 Tbsp. Dijon-style mustard

Whisk together ingredients in a small bowl. Pour over chicken and turn to coat.

NUTRITION FACTS
(¼-cup serving):
23 calories, 0 g protein, 1 g carbs, 0 g fat

3) Hot 'n' Tangy Marinade

>> ¼ cup cider vinegar
>> ¼ cup ketchup
>> ¼ cup fresh lemon juice
>> 2 Tbsp. nonhydrogenated margarine, melted
>> 2 Tbsp. prepared horseradish
>> 1 tsp. Worcestershire sauce
>> Few drops of hot sauce

Combine ingredients in a small pan and bring to a boil. Lower heat, cover and simmer for 10 minutes. Pour over chicken and turn to coat.

NUTRITION FACTS
(¼-cup serving):
29 calories, 0 g protein, 8 g carbs, 1 g fat

4) Spicy Dry Rub

>> ½ Tbsp. paprika
>> ½ tsp. brown sugar
>> ½ tsp. coarse salt
>> ½ tsp. ground pepper
>> ¼ tsp. dried thyme
>> ¼ tsp. cayenne pepper

Stir together ingredients in a small bowl. Rub into chicken before cooking.

and since you're paying by weight, you're actually paying for this H$_2$O. And although there's no nutritional difference between organic and regular chicken, you'll avoid ingesting antibiotics and hormones when you buy certified organic poultry.

BE A PRO: Free-range chicken is already at a flavor advantage, so why overpower it with a lot of external flavors? "I tend to rub only kosher salt and pepper onto high-end breasts," says chef Hinnerk von Bargen, associate professor at the Culinary Institute of America (Hyde Park, New York; St. Helena, California). "Sometimes less really is more."

RULE #2: Give It a Bath

Marinating is the best way to overcome chicken's rather bland natural flavor. "Marinades keep chicken from drying out and make it more exciting," says Brennan. He recommends marinating chicken breasts for at least eight hours in the refrigerator to infuse more flavor, and set aside a little extra for basting during cooking.

Basic marinades include an acid such as vinegar, wine or citrus juice along with oil and spice and herb flavorings. But why stop there? Try our marinades and rub in "Fowl Play" (above) for new ways to perk up your poultry.

BE A PRO: Freeze chicken breasts in a zip-top bag with your marinade. The breast will soak it in as it defrosts.

RULE #3: Rub Your Bird

No time to wait for your breast to marinate? Try a rub! Like a marinade, a rub — basically a blend of salt, spices and herbs — can be just the right touch to make chicken taste great. "A bit of coarse salt mixed with cumin and

FAST FOOD FIX

BETWEEN THE 9-TO-5 GRIND, PUMPING IRON AND WATCHING THE BIG GAME, YOU MIGHT RESORT TO THE DRIVE-THRU PIT STOP. MOST FAST-FOOD CHICKEN IS HIGHER IN FAT, CALORIES AND SODIUM THAN WHAT YOU'D MAKE AT HOME, BUT WITH A LITTLE NUTRITIONAL SAVVY, YOU CAN GET AWAY WITH CATCHING YOUR BIRD ON THE FLY.

YOU WIN

>> KFC Tender Roast Sandwich, no sauce (217 g): 300 calories, 37 g protein, 23 g carbs, 5 g fat (1.5 g sat, 0 g trans), 1,060 mg sodium

>> McDonald's Premium Grilled Chicken Classic Sandwich (229 g): 420 calories, 32 g protein, 51 g carbs, 10 g fat (2 g sat, 0 g trans), 1,190 mg sodium

>> Subway 12-inch Oven Roast Chicken Breast (474 g): 670 calories, 43 g protein, 95 g carbs, 11 g fat (7 g sat, 0 g trans), 1,680 mg sodium
Note: To cut down on the carbs and total calories, ditch half of the bread and stack the extra chicken on the other side.

YOU LOSE

>> KFC Large Popcorn Chicken (160 g): 550 calories, 29 g protein, 30 g carbs, 35 g fat (6 g sat, 0 g trans), 1,600 mg sodium

>> McDonald's Premium Crispy Chicken Club Sandwich (250 g): 530 calories, 36 g protein, 60 g carbs, 28 g fat (7 g sat, 0 g trans), 1,420 mg sodium

>> Subway 6-inch Chicken & Bacon Ranch (298 g): 580 calories, 36 g protein, 47 g carbs, 30 g fat (11 g sat, 1 g trans), 1,390 mg sodium

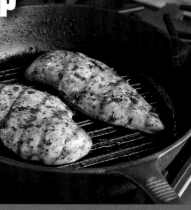

Grill-Top
Chicken Breasts

>> Coat a grill pan with cooking spray and preheat over medium heat. Cook marinated breasts 5–6 minutes per side or until cooked thoroughly. You can also use an outdoor grill.

4 SAMPLE MEALS

With Hot 'n' Tangy Marinade >> 6 oz. chicken breast >> 2 medium baked sweet potatoes >> 1 cup mixed vegetables	**NUTRITION FACTS*** 557 calories, 49 g protein, 87 g carbs, 3 g fat
With Tandoori Marinade >> 6 oz. chicken breast >> 1½ cups cooked lentils >> 2 cups green salad >> 2 Tbsp. fat-free Italian dressing	**NUTRITION FACTS*** 610 calories, 70 g protein, 74 g carbs, 4 g fat
With Red Wine Marinade >> 6 oz. chicken breast >> 1½ cups cooked wild rice >> 1 can French cut green beans	**NUTRITION FACTS*** 508 calories, 53 g protein, 64 g carbs, 3 g fat
With Spicy Dry Rub >> 6 oz. chicken breast >> ½ cup kidney beans >> 1 cup cooked long-grain white rice >> 1 cup cooked okra	**NUTRITION FACTS** 551 calories, 56 g protein, 73 g carbs, 3 g fat * Totals include marinade values

turmeric or oregano and garlic are among my favorite spices to rub into chicken," says von Bargen.

Other common rub ingredients include dry mustard, chili powder, rosemary, ground coriander, cayenne and paprika. "For added taste, I like squirting on some lemon juice toward the end of cooking a seasoned breast," von Bargen adds. An acid ingredient like lemon or other citrus juice can stimulate your taste buds so less salt is needed.

BE A PRO: Before rubbing in your seasonings, add a few drops of oil to the chicken to help the rub stick.

RULE #4: Don't Overcook — or Undercook

Overcooking chicken can ruin the taste, but undercooking is even worse, as it can leave you kneeling over the porcelain throne. To get around this problem, use a cooking thermometer to determine when your breasts are cooked just right.

"Chicken breast should be cooked to an internal temperature of 165 degrees F," von Bargen explains. This will annihilate those nasty bugs while keeping your chicken moist.

BE A PRO: Let your chicken rest for a few minutes after cooking is complete. "This allows the juices to redistribute moisture throughout the meat, which adds flavor," advises Brennan.

RULE #5: Try a Brine

A surefire way to avoid dry breasts is to soak them in brine. "I love brining because the salt and water penetrate the chicken, which makes it moist," says von Bargen.

Basic brine consists of 1 tablespoon of salt added to each cup of water used. Enough water should be added to submerge the chicken. "Like marinating, a good brining takes overnight," von Bargen adds. If you're time-strapped, frozen breasts can be left to defrost in brine. But keep in mind that brined chicken will cook faster because water is a heat conductor.

BE A PRO: There's no reason to stop at salt. "Add herbs, spices and juices to brining water to really make things interesting," von Bargen points out.

FACT

85

>> percent of calories in a 6-ounce chicken breast come from protein

RULE #6: Pack and Store It

While nothing matches the taste of fresh-cooked chicken, grilling several breasts at once is more convenient for time-starved trainees. But keeping cooked chicken in the fridge longer than three days is risky, so use your freezer for leftovers. A vacuum sealer can stamp out freezer burn and extend a chicken's frozen life. Just make sure you don't extend it too long — chicken frozen longer than four months should be thrown out.

When cooking and storing chicken in batches, cool and refrigerate (or freeze) it within two hours. Don't store it while it's still hot. Use airtight containers to prevent chicken from drying out, losing nutritional value and taking on surrounding refrigerator flavors, von Bargen advises. When it comes to reheating leftovers in the microwave, "use a low heat setting and cover the dish; both retain moisture and flavor," he explains. Adding a little broth or water also helps.

BE A PRO: Brining leftover cooked chicken will make it juicy again.

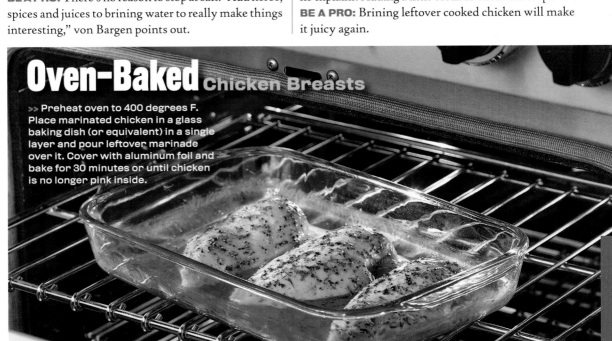

Oven-Baked Chicken Breasts

>> Preheat oven to 400 degrees F. Place marinated chicken in a glass baking dish (or equivalent) in a single layer and pour leftover marinade over it. Cover with aluminum foil and bake for 30 minutes or until chicken is no longer pink inside.

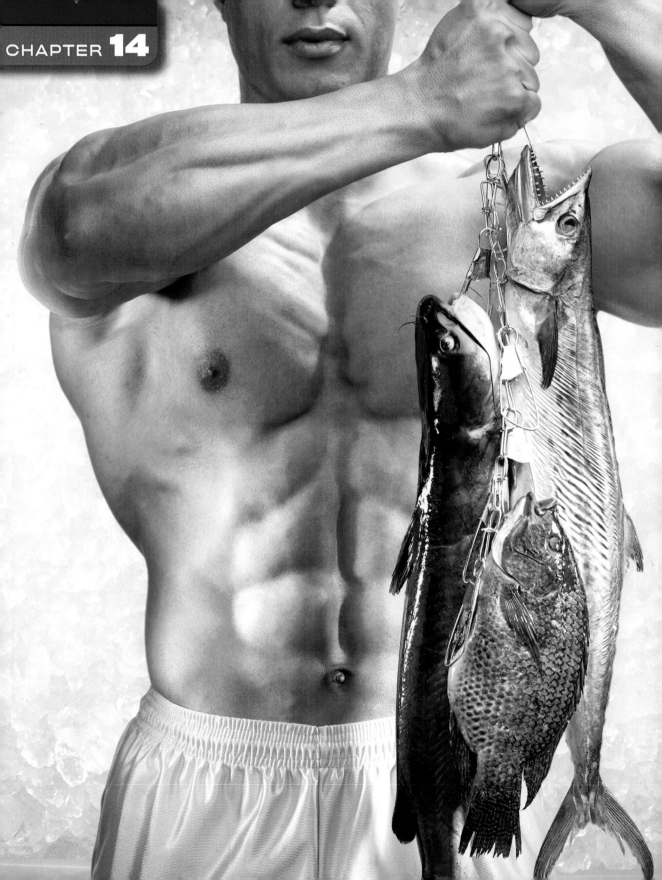

Reel In The Gains

Back in the 1970s, scientists ventured to Greenland to study the lifestyle of the Inuit people. Despite their lack of vegetables, fruits and whole grains — foods we've been led to believe are dietary musts — the Inuits were remarkably healthy, with strong hearts and sturdy joints. Their dietary secret? They were fueled by impressive amounts of fatty sea life!

This discovery doesn't necessarily mean we should give up our current nutritional habits and all eat like an Intuit. But it is a good lesson on why fish should be a regular part of a healthy diet. Too often, bodybuilders concerned about getting enough high-quality protein reach first for the cow, hog or bird, leaving fish to flounder in their nutritional regimens.

But fish should be front and center in any bodybuilding diet because it's loaded with protein, the world's healthiest fats and assorted other great nutrients. Just make sure it's not battered and fried — those are cooking methods that scuttle the health benefits and send them to the bottom.

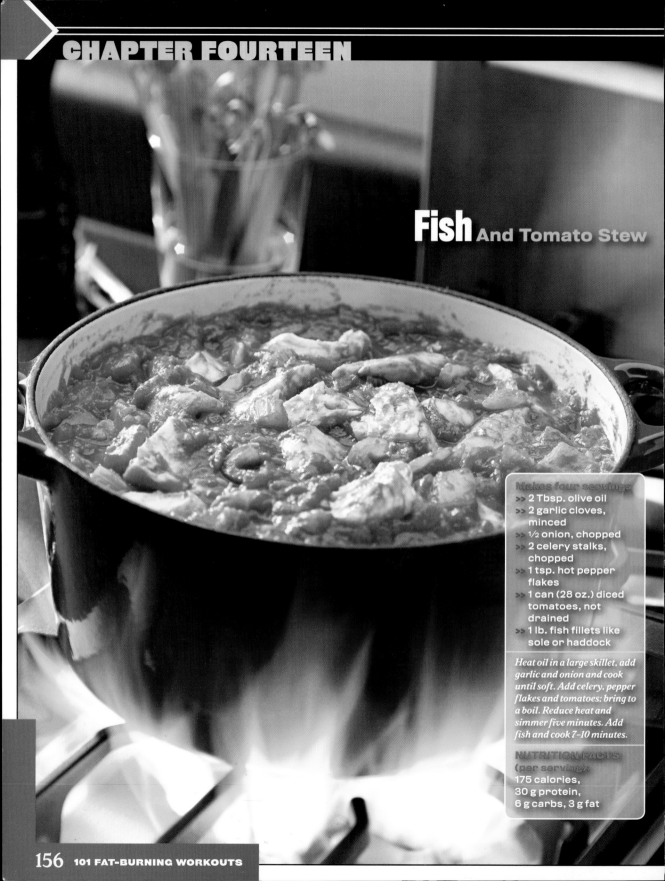

Fish And Tomato Stew

Makes four servings

>> 2 Tbsp. olive oil
>> 2 garlic cloves, minced
>> ½ onion, chopped
>> 2 celery stalks, chopped
>> 1 tsp. hot pepper flakes
>> 1 can (28 oz.) diced tomatoes, not drained
>> 1 lb. fish fillets like sole or haddock

Heat oil in a large skillet, add garlic and onion and cook until soft. Add celery, pepper flakes and tomatoes; bring to a boil. Reduce heat and simmer five minutes. Add fish and cook 7–10 minutes.

NUTRITION FACTS (per serving):
175 calories,
30 g protein,
6 g carbs, 3 g fat

Loaded with protein, fish should be the centerpiece of any bodybuilder's diet — as long as you know how to reel in the right kind.

OMEGA POWER

When it comes to beef, chicken and pork, you've heard it before: Cut the fat. Well, throw out that advice for fish, because the fattier, the better. The predominant fat in fish is the type that will keep your arteries sparkling clean.

Fatty fish like salmon, sardines and mackerel are the only reliable dietary sources of eicosapentanoic acid (EPA) and docosohexanoic acid (DHA), two potent omega-3 fatty acids with a broad range of health benefits. "By reducing inflammation and the stickiness of the blood and lowering triglyceride levels, fish fat is very heart-protective," states Monique Ryan, MS, RD, a sports dietitian and author of *Performance Nutrition for Team Sports* (Peak Sports Press, 2005). Because it's involved in pathways that reduce inflammation, fish fat may also help minimize muscle irritation associated with killer workouts.

While omega-3 fatty acids' role in heart health is now well established, what gets little play in the media is their potential to help shed bodyfat. It's true: By altering gene regulation, DHA and EPA have the means to accelerate fat-burning via increased enzyme activity for fat oxidation. DHA's

FISH COOKING 101

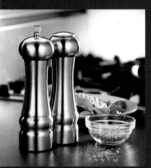

It's a real heartbreak when you buy the perfect cut of fish only to have it turn out drier than Death Valley. But with some simple precautions from Richard Chamberlain, chef and owner of Chamberlain's Fish Market Grill in Dallas, your fish cooking experience doesn't need to have a tragic ending.

» START FRESH A truly fresh cut of seafood should be very shiny with bright colors. A smell test also works: A good fillet will have no odor. Reputable fish markets like Whole Foods are your best bet for the good stuff.

» BE GENTLE Handle your fish as little as possible. Let it cook undisturbed for a few minutes, and turn only once during cooking. "This allows for carmelization (browning) of proteins on the surface, which contributes to the flavor. When the color at the sides of the fish becomes pale, it's time to flip."

» ADD FLAVOR Simplicity pays off when it comes to fish. "A salt-and-pepper rub using a good-quality sea salt is all a really good steak or fillet needs." A rule of thumb is three parts sea salt to one part freshly ground pepper. If you marinate it, do so for only 30 minutes. "Fish is more tender and porous than most meats, so it needs less time in a marinade."

» DON'T OVERCOOK Delicate fish like sole and flounder cook quickly, about two minutes per side if sautéing, grilling or broiling. For thicker fish like salmon, swordfish and sea bass, "Just as the color changes from translucent to opaque, remove from heat and serve immediately." Avoid cooking fish until it flakes easily, which makes it dry.

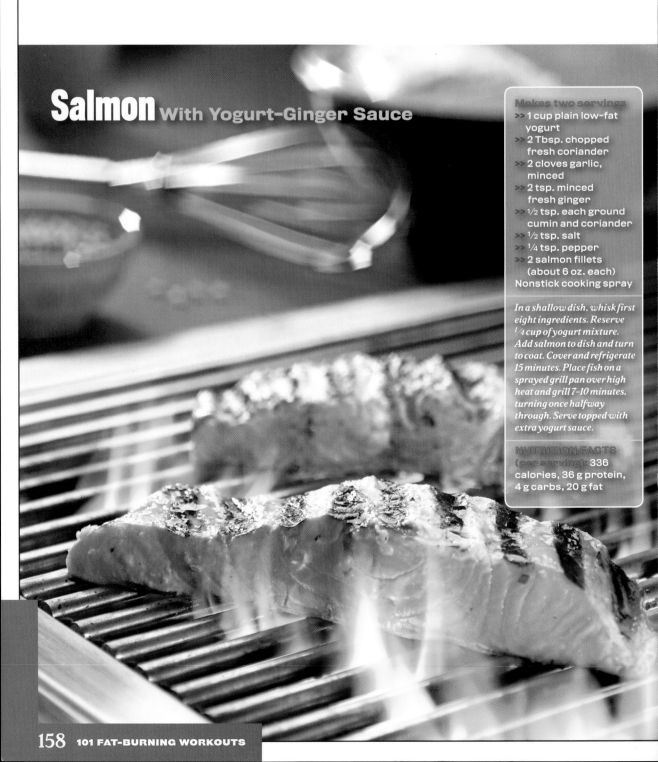

Salmon With Yogurt-Ginger Sauce

Makes two servings
>> 1 cup plain low-fat yogurt
>> 2 Tbsp. chopped fresh coriander
>> 2 cloves garlic, minced
>> 2 tsp. minced fresh ginger
>> 1/2 tsp. each ground cumin and coriander
>> 1/2 tsp. salt
>> 1/4 tsp. pepper
>> 2 salmon fillets (about 6 oz. each)
Nonstick cooking spray

In a shallow dish, whisk first eight ingredients. Reserve 1/4 cup of yogurt mixture. Add salmon to dish and turn to coat. Cover and refrigerate 15 minutes. Place fish on a sprayed grill pan over high heat and grill 7–10 minutes, turning once halfway through. Serve topped with extra yogurt sauce.

NUTRITION FACTS (per serving): 336 calories, 36 g protein, 4 g carbs, 20 g fat ability to improve insulin sensitivity will also keep the jiggle at bay by improving sugar and protein metabolism. And let's not overlook that it may keep men more fertile. Yes, it truly is the wonder fat.

PROTEIN PUNCH

Since muscles are made of protein, obviously you'd make sure to eat enough of it if you wanted arms like a pro bodybuilder. Where better to start than with a gift from the sea? "Most fish is a lean protein source," says Ryan. It has an excellent protein-to-fat ratio, which will keep you in an anabolic state — key to muscle growth. It's also a good whole-food protein to eat before and after workouts; compared to beef, pork and poultry, fish is digested and absorbed faster. "Fish's amino acid profile also makes it especially useful in repairing and building muscles," Ryan explains.

THE LITTLE GUYS

Even though the omega-3s and protein get all the accolades when it comes to seafood, there's other stuff under those gills that'll keep you out of the doctor's office and on the gym floor. The iron in fish helps carry oxygen to your working muscles; vitamin B_6 assists in red-blood-cell formation; and selenium can keep your prostate in good working order by preventing oxidative damage as well as support thyroid function, critical for keeping your metabolism in check.

FACT

500

>> Approximate amount (in mg) of omega-3s in a 1,000-mg capsule of fish oil

And after spending an evening at the oyster bar, you'll have had enough zinc to boost those testosterone levels.

FISHING FOR MERCURY

But if you're not careful, you could end up eating fish with more heavy metal than a Metallica album. Although most of the warnings regarding mercury in seafood focus on children and pregnant women, even the mightiest men need to beware of this powerful neurotoxin.

"A general rule of thumb is that larger fish like shark, swordfish, tuna and king mackerel — and those that tend to stick around for a long time such as orange roughy, grouper, Chilean sea bass and Pacific rock bass — can accumulate lots of mercury," reports Timothy Fitzgerald, Environmental Defense researcher. There are no specific guidelines for males when it comes to consumption, but Fitzgerald recommends that men eat these fish only occasionally and instead focus on those with lower levels of mercury. (The American Heart Association recommends at least two 3-ounce servings of fish a week, but no more than 12 ounces.) "Wild salmon, catfish, shellfish, Pacific halibut, sardines, small mackerel, tilapia and rainbow trout are safer options," Fitzgerald notes. Visit oceansalive.org for an extensive listing of the fish that are safe to reel in on your dinner plate.

As for that proverbial bodybuilding staple, canned tuna, albacore "solid white" tuna has roughly three times more mercury than "chunk light" tuna. "Albacore is a much larger fish than the skipjack used mostly for light tuna," says Fitzgerald. So if you're devouring several cans of tuna a week, make sure to stick with the cheaper stuff or, better yet, switch to canned salmon, which is not only lower in mercury but also higher in omega-3s.

> **Fish has an excellent protein-to-fat ratio, which will keep you in an anabolic state — key to muscle growth.**

Halibut With Lemon-Mustard Sauce

Makes two servings
- >> ¼ cup lemon juice
- >> ½ Tbsp. lemon zest
- >> 2 Tbsp. Dijon mustard
- >> 1 Tbsp. dried tarragon
- >> 1 scallion, chopped
- >> ¼ tsp. pepper
- >> 2 Tbsp. olive oil
- >> 2 halibut fillets (about 6 oz. each)

Nonstick cooking spray

Combine first six ingredients in a shallow dish. Slowly stir in oil and whisk well. Add halibut and turn to coat. Cover and refrigerate 30 minutes. Place fish on a sprayed grill pan over high heat and grill 5–7 minutes per side.

NUTRITION FACTS (per serving):
269 calories, 33 g protein, 4 g carbs, 10 g fat

UNDER THE SEA

You've been diligently downing cans of tuna to meet your daily protein quota, but now you're ready to dive into deeper waters and try something new. Before you head to the sushi bar or your local fishmonger at the grocery store, check out our guide to help you choose the best fish for your physique.

FISH (6 OZ. COOKED)	CALORIES	PROTEIN (G)	FAT (G)	OMEGA-3S (G)
1) Mackerel, mixed species	342	44	17	3.4
2) Herring	345	40	20	3.5
3) Salmon, Atlantic, farmed	350	38	21	3.6
4) Salmon, Chinook	392	44	22	3.5
5) Salmon, Sockeye	368	46	18	2.4
6) Salmon, canned, pink	232	40	8	2
7) Sardines, canned	354	42	20	1
8) Shark	260	42	10	1.8
9) Trout	324	46	14	2
10) Tuna, canned, white	218	40	5	1.4
11) Swordfish	264	43	9	1.4
12) Sea Bass	210	40	4	1.4
13) Halibut	238	45	5	1
14) Crab, blue	173	34	3	1
15) Lobster, spiny	243	45	3	1
16) Tuna, fresh or frozen	236	51	2	0.5
17) Oysters, Pacific	278	32	8	2.4
18) Tuna, canned, light	197	43	1	0.5
19) Shrimp	168	36	2	0.6
20) Haddock	190	41	1.6	0.4
21) Catfish	258	32	14	0.4
22) Tilapia	218	44	5	0.4
23) Cod, Atlantic	178	39	2	0.3
24) Mahi Mahi	186	40	2	0.2

source: nal.usda.gov/fnic/foodcomp/cgi-bin/

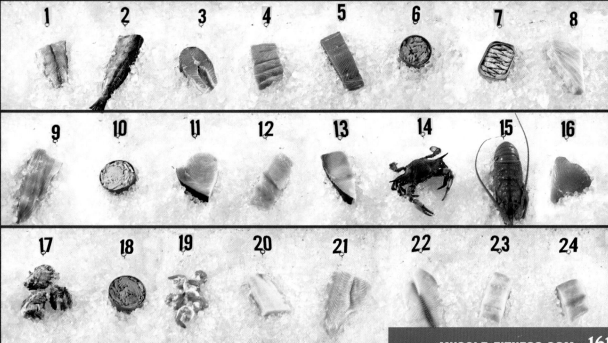

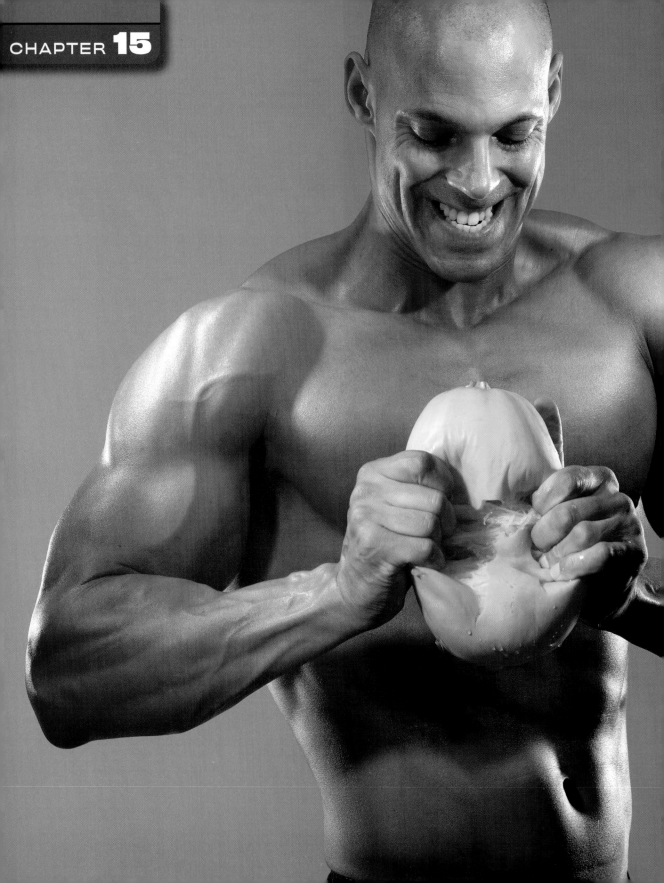

Crunch-Time Salads

Are you a guy who scoffs at the mere thought of giving up your beloved protein for a big bowl of lettuce, carrots, peppers, tomatoes and cucumber slices? Big mistake!

You need your veggies if you want to reach your full muscle-building potential. Lauded by health experts, doctors and your mom (remember her saying, "You're not getting any dessert until you eat all your broccoli"?), vegetables don't have a sexy rep, but their therapeutic and healing properties are essential to keeping you as healthy as possible for maximum gym efforts. And a bodybuilder in optimal health will make gains faster than one who isn't.

So ignore vegetables at your body's peril. This chapter contains all the information you need on why veggies are a must, along with what produce is best to keep in the crisper.

CHAPTER FIFTEEN

VEGGING OUT

From fighting disease to revealing your washboard abs, there are so many reasons to spend more time in the produce aisle that we could fill an entire book. These are the most important reasons to say, "More, please," when it comes to vegetables.

MIGHTY PHYTOS Unlike fiber and vitamins, what you don't see in those vegetable nutrition charts are the powerhouse antioxidant chemicals called phytochemicals. A vegetable will produce them to protect itself during growth, but many phytochemicals, such as lycopene in tomatoes and carotenoids in carrots, can also protect us against many ailments. There's even a group of phytochemicals called indoles (found in cruciferous vegetables, such as cabbage and broccoli) that stimulate enzymes to make estrogen less effective — a definite advantage if you yearn for more mass. Acting as antioxidants, phytochemicals also aid in postworkout muscle repair.

BULKING UP Vegetables are a great source of something often neglected in bodybuilding nutrition — fiber. As a source of bulk, veggies can slow digestion,

A BETTER SALAD

GO WITH A VARIETY OF COLOR. DEEPLY HUED VEGGIES REIGN SUPREME WHEN IT COMES TO DISEASE-FIGHTING, IMMUNE-BOOSTING CHEMICALS.

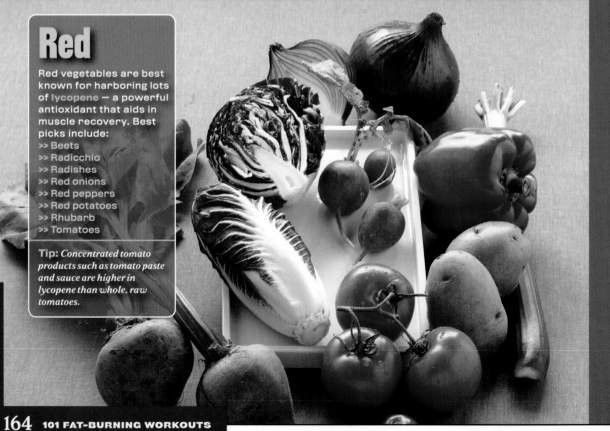

Red

Red vegetables are best known for harboring lots of lycopene — a powerful antioxidant that aids in muscle recovery. Best picks include:

>> Beets
>> Radicchio
>> Radishes
>> Red onions
>> Red peppers
>> Red potatoes
>> Rhubarb
>> Tomatoes

Tip: Concentrated tomato products such as tomato paste and sauce are higher in lycopene than whole, raw tomatoes.

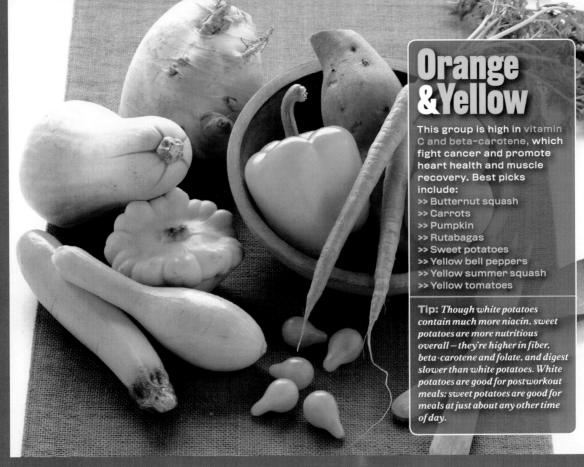

Orange & Yellow

This group is high in vitamin C and beta-carotene, which fight cancer and promote heart health and muscle recovery. Best picks include:

>> Butternut squash
>> Carrots
>> Pumpkin
>> Rutabagas
>> Sweet potatoes
>> Yellow bell peppers
>> Yellow summer squash
>> Yellow tomatoes

Tip: *Though white potatoes contain much more niacin, sweet potatoes are more nutritious overall — they're higher in fiber, beta-carotene and folate, and digest slower than white potatoes. White potatoes are good for postworkout meals; sweet potatoes are good for meals at just about any other time of day.*

which helps regulate blood-sugar levels. Spikes in blood sugar (which often come from eating high-carbohydrate, low-fiber foods like white bread) promote fat storage, and sudden drops can cause energy "crashes," making it less likely that you'll push serious weight at the gym. Add vegetables to your lunchtime stir-fry and you could say *adios* to those ups and downs. You'll also tend to eat less because low-calorie, higher-fiber veggies take up room in the stomach and release chemicals that tell the brain to shut down the appetite. And don't overlook the fact that by improving digestion, fiber can support the absorption of vitamins, minerals and amino acids — all of which your muscles need for further growth.

BURN, BABY, BURN Vegetables are a "free food" with a very low calorie-density, so you can eat almost unlimited amounts while still burning fat. This lean indulgence is all because of a biochemical quirk that only veggies (except the starchier ones like corn and beets) enjoy — the body uses almost as many calories to digest vegetables as they contain in the first place. The leftover calories don't even have a fighting chance of being stored in a fat cell.

VEGETABLES 101

Filling your grocery cart with more vegetables is only half the battle — you also need to know what to do with them once you get home. This can sometimes be more challenging than developing arms like a bodybuilding pro, so let us help.

FACT

400

>> mcg is the recommended daily intake for folate

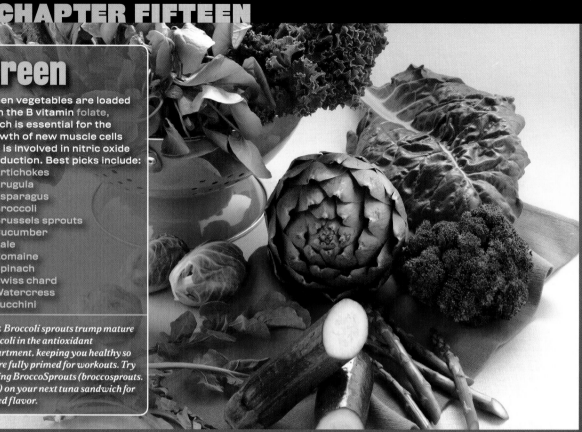

Green

Green vegetables are loaded with the B vitamin folate, which is essential for the growth of new muscle cells and is involved in nitric oxide production. Best picks include:

>> Artichokes
>> Arugula
>> Asparagus
>> Broccoli
>> Brussels sprouts
>> Cucumber
>> Kale
>> Romaine
>> Spinach
>> Swiss chard
>> Watercress
>> Zucchini

Tip: *Broccoli sprouts trump mature broccoli in the antioxidant department. keeping you healthy so you're fully primed for workouts. Try tossing BroccoSprouts (broccosprouts. com) on your next tuna sandwich for added flavor.*

White

Allicin, a phytochemical found in the onion family, is stellar at maintaining healthy testosterone levels and inhibiting cortisol production. It also helps prevent cardiovascular disease. Best picks include:

>> Cauliflower
>> Garlic
>> Jicama
>> Mushrooms
>> Onions
>> Parsnips
>> Shallots
>> Turnips
>> White potatoes

Tip: *To get the most out of allicin-containing foods such as garlic and onions, don't heat them for too long — this chemical is very heat-sensitive and will break down easily.*

SELECTION "Seek out vegetables that are at their peak ripeness," says Cathy Thomas, a food editor for the *Orange County Register*, a newspaper in Southern California. Ripeness varies, but as a rule, avoid leafy greens that are wilting and firmer produce such as peppers and zucchini that have soft spots and discoloration.

"Peak produce has more nutrient content than overripe or underripe versions," Thomas advises. Usually farmers' markets will have the best selection of perfectly ripe vegetables.

STORAGE Because flavors and textures are at their peak right after picking, the best advice is to shop often and store fresh vegetables for only 2–3 days.

"Different veggies prefer different storage situations," says Thomas. "Some, such as salad greens, prefer the fridge, while others, such as artichokes and tomatoes, respond more favorably to the counter." Check out Thomas' book, *Melissa's Great Book of Produce* (Wiley, 2006) for proper storage techniques for every imaginable vegetable.

COOKING When it comes to moving vegetables beyond their raw state, your goal should be to preserve as much of their nutrients as possible. Contact with boiling water can cause water-soluble nutrients such as B vitamins and vitamin C to leach out into the water. Steaming is best for preserving nutrients since there's no direct water contact and the temperature is more moderate. The microwave and the high heat of a frying pan can damage some nutrients, but tomatoes, corn and carrots are actually more nutritious when slightly cooked.

FRESH VS. FROZEN If you can be sure that the fresh vegetables are indeed fresh, that would be the most nutritious choice. The longer a "fresh" vegetable travels across the country or sits in the store, however, the less nutritious it becomes. That's why frozen-food processors "flash-freeze" their vegetables as soon as they're picked, thus preserving most of their vitamins. This makes those bags of frozen mixed vegetables a nutritious option when you're in a rush. To preserve nutrients, steam, don't boil, your frozen delights.

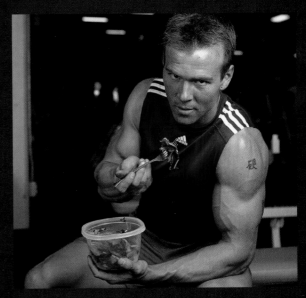

WORKOUT VEGGIES

OF COURSE WE ALWAYS RECOMMEND A PRE- AND POSTWORKOUT PROTEIN SHAKE, BUT THE LAST WHOLE-FOOD MEAL YOU EAT BEFORE YOUR WORKOUT AND THE FIRST ONE YOU EAT AFTER YOU TRAIN SHOULD CONTAIN CERTAIN VEGETABLES.

PREWORKOUT, eat a salad with your meal. Research shows that the phytochemicals in salad can help boost nitric oxide production and increase blood flow to exercising muscles. Salad greens that are darker in color — think romaine, watercress and arugula — provide more nutritional benefits; the old standby, iceberg lettuce, doesn't contain much more than water.

POSTWORKOUT, your meal should contain onions and broccoli. Onions contain the compound allyl propyl disulfide, which increases insulin levels. This is the one time you want a boost in insulin levels because the hormone drives carbs and creatine into your muscles. It also stimulates muscle protein synthesis, the process of muscle growth. Broccoli contains chromium, an essential trace mineral that enhances insulin's effects on muscle cells.

INDEX OF EXERCISES

Below is a listing of exercises broken down by bodypart; if listed here, the movement is described, and in most cases pictured, on the listed page.

101 FAT-BURNING WORKOUT CHART

MONDAY EXERCISE	SET 1 REPS / WEIGHT		SET 2 REPS / WEIGHT		SET 3 REPS / WEIGHT		SET 4 REPS / WEIGHT		SET 5 REPS / WEIGHT	

TUESDAY EXERCISE	SET 1 REPS / WEIGHT		SET 2 REPS / WEIGHT		SET 3 REPS / WEIGHT		SET 4 REPS / WEIGHT		SET 5 REPS / WEIGHT	

WEDNESDAY EXERCISE	SET 1 REPS / WEIGHT		SET 2 REPS / WEIGHT		SET 3 REPS / WEIGHT		SET 4 REPS / WEIGHT		SET 5 REPS / WEIGHT	

THURSDAY EXERCISE	SET 1 REPS / WEIGHT		SET 2 REPS / WEIGHT		SET 3 REPS / WEIGHT		SET 4 REPS / WEIGHT		SET 5 REPS / WEIGHT	

101 FAT-BURNING WORKOUT CHART

FRIDAY EXERCISE	SET 1 REPS / WEIGHT	SET 2 REPS / WEIGHT	SET 3 REPS / WEIGHT	SET 4 REPS / WEIGHT	SET 5 REPS / WEIGHT

SATURDAY EXERCISE	SET 1 REPS / WEIGHT	SET 2 REPS / WEIGHT	SET 3 REPS / WEIGHT	SET 4 REPS / WEIGHT	SET 5 REPS / WEIGHT

SUNDAY EXERCISE	SET 1 REPS / WEIGHT	SET 2 REPS / WEIGHT	SET 3 REPS / WEIGHT	SET 4 REPS / WEIGHT	SET 5 REPS / WEIGHT

CARDIO	EXERCISE	TIME	NOTES
MONDAY			
TUESDAY			
WEDNESDAY			
THURSDAY			
FRIDAY			
SATURDAY			
SUNDAY			

MEALS

DATE:

QUANTITY	FOOD/LIQUIDS/SUPPLEMENTS	TIME	CALORIES	PROTEIN	CARBS	FAT
	TOTALS					

LIQUIDS: 8 OZ = 1 CUP | 4 CUPS = 1 QUART | 4 QUARTS = 1 GALLON
WEIGHT: 16 OZ = 1 LB | 1 LB = 454 GRAMS | 1 OZ = 28.35 GRAMS

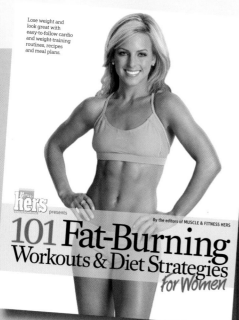
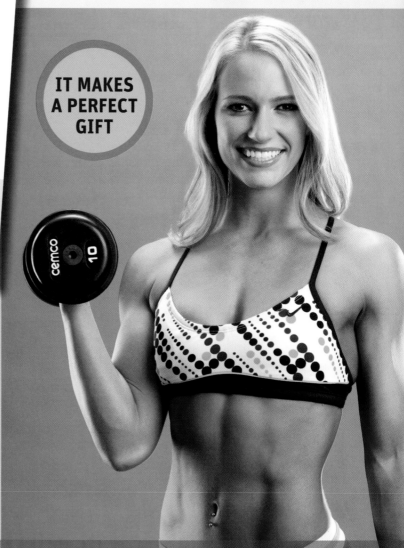